# Access to Health and Education Services in Ethiopia

## Supply, Demand, and Government Policy

Fra von Massow

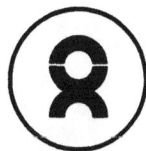

**Oxfam**

First published by Oxfam GB in 2001
This edition transferred to print-on-demand in 2007

© Oxfam GB 2001

ISBN 0 85598 471 6

Available from:
Bournemouth English Book Centre, PO Box 1496, Parkstone, Dorset, BH12 3YD, UK
tel: +44 (0)1202 712933; fax: +44 (0)1202 712930; email: oxfam@bebc.co.uk

USA: Stylus Publishing LLC, PO Box 605, Herndon, VA 20172-0605, USA
tel: +1 (0)703 661 1581; fax: +1 (0)703 661 1547; email: styluspub@aol.com

For details of local agents and representatives in other countries, consult our website: www.oxfam.org.uk/publications
or contact Oxfam Publishing, Oxfam House, John Smith Drive, Cowley, Oxford, OX4 2JY, UK
tel +44 (0) 1865 472255; fax (0) 1865 472393; email: publish@oxfam.org.uk

Our website contains a fully searchable database of all our titles, and facilities for secure on-line ordering.

Published by Oxfam GB, Oxfam House, John Smith Drive, Cowley, Oxford, OX4 2JY, UK

Oxfam GB is a registered charity, no. 202918, and is a member of Oxfam International.

# Contents

# Acknowledgements

This summary report gives me the opportunity to express my high regard for the members of the team who conducted the field studies on which it is based. It was a very bright, energetic, and tireless group of individuals, men and women of mixed ages and experience. There was a strong sense of devotion to the task and a spirit of co-operation and support for one another throughout the three months in which we lived and worked together. The team included Almaz Terefe (Senior Researcher, Health), Dr Abebe Bekele (Senior Researcher, Education); Assistant Researchers Tsehay Haile, Amare Worku, Awet Kidane Gebrehiwot, and Taddesse Koyra; Senior Statistician Samuel Feyissa; and Damenech Zewdi (Logistics Co-ordinator and Secretary). We were supported by Zerfi Zerehoun and accompanied by Worku Taddesse and Berhane Gebre Egziabher: two excellent drivers assigned to us by Oxfam.

The research was launched with the guidance and support of Dr Mohga Smith from Oxfam's Policy Department in Oxford. Her input was much appreciated by the whole team. Othman Mohamed, then Oxfam's Ethiopia Director, awarded the research high priority throughout and put staff and facilities at the team's disposal. The team's endeavours were at all times supported by the Oxfam staff in Addis Ababa, who were extremely accommodating, friendly, and helpful, despite the huge demands on their time. The Oxfam block managers gave the team advice and support whenever it was required. In Addis Ababa the team could not have done its work in the first site without the daily support and assistance of the staff of the Voluntary Centre for the Handicapped. In the regions we were guided and assisted by the Oxfam staff in the regional offices in Dessie, Wogel Tena, Delanta, Deder, Eastern Hararge, and Jijiga, Somali Region. They organised our accommodation and food, and they looked after our personal needs. They made all preparations for the research, including briefing the team and preparing the community, and they accompanied us in the field. The team developed a strong appreciation for the high calibre and devotion to their work of the Oxfam field staff, who live and work in extremely difficult circumstances. In Deder and Jijiga the team was additionally assisted by excellent translators, kindly assigned by the respective government offices for health and education.

In each site visited, the team met with first-level health and education service providers: teachers, school directors, health assistants, and directors; and with local authorities. We were often overwhelmed by the time that they spared and the hospitality that they accorded to us. Many are devoted professionals, working in remote locations with the absolute minimum of resources, in conditions of extreme deprivation. Traditional practitioners shared their wealth of experience and their difficulties with the team.

Nor would the research have been possible without the co-operation and time given by women, men, and young girls and boys, in Cherkos, Addis Ababa; Yegurassa and Andaje villages in North Wollo; Ali Roba village in Eastern Hararge; and Belhare and Sheik Umer villages in Somali region. This summary report is dedicated to them. It aims to reflect as closely as possible the reality of poverty, hunger, and deprivation which they described to us and with which they have to cope every day. It is the team's strongest wish that these reports might influence decision makers at local, national, and international levels in the interests of reducing poverty and increasing access to good-quality basic health services and reproductive-health services for all, and elementary education for all school-age children. To this end the team's families and friends in Addis Ababa and London provided the necessary support to facilitate the work.

The research into national policies and economic trends was carried out by Dr Abdulhamid Bedri Kello and Mr Getachew Yoseph.

For their insights and support I am indebted to all the contributors named above; but the recommendations contained in this paper, and the integrated analysis of the field-study findings and the macro-economic data, are my sole responsibility.

*Fra von Massow*
*Research team leader*

# Glossary

| | |
|---|---|
| *Almaze* | a skin disease which can become acute |
| **ANC** | antenatal clinic |
| *Ato* | the term used for 'Mr' |
| *Baldi* | a bucket with a capacity of 20 litres |
| *Bega* | the dry or sunny season |
| *berberri* | hot pepper spice |
| *birrd* | a generic term for colds, rheumatism, and chest problems |
| **bonesetter** | a traditional physiotherapist who specialises in fractures |
| *buna bet* | coffee shop |
| *'chat* | an addictive stimulant, consumed mostly by men, who chew the leaves of this plant |
| *damakesse* | a herb commonly used for practically all types of ailments |
| *debtera* | a churchman, trained for the priesthood, who treats the sick by writing some script on a piece of paper and scrolling it into a very small piece, which is then sewn into a small piece of cloth to make it into a charm that the sick person wears on his/her neck by suspending it on a piece of thread. The *debtera* is believed to have the ability to make somebody sick by using the same ritual. |
| *Derg* | the commonly used name for the regime of Mengistu Haile Mariam which ruled Ethiopia following a popular revolution which unseated the government of Emperor Haile Selassie in 1974 |
| **DPPC** | Disaster Prevention and Preparedness Committee |
| **EC** | Ethiopian Calendar |
| **ENT** | ear, nose, and throat |
| **EPI** | extended programme for immunisation |
| **EPRDF** | Ethiopian People's Revolutionary Democratic Front |
| **FGD** | focus-group discussions |
| **FGM** | female genital mutilation |
| **FP** | family planning |
| *Ginbot* | May |
| *gote* | a village of 70-100 households. There are between five and eight *gotes* in one Peasant Association |
| *Hamiley* | July |
| *Harafar* | a Muslim holy day |
| *Hidar* | November |
| *idir* | a community savings club for the eventuality of a death or marriage in the community |
| **IEC** | Information, Education, and Communication |
| *injera* | a national staple: a flat pancake made with *teff* (a local grain), barley, or sorghum. It is typically eaten with a spicy sauce or stew. |
| *Kebele* | the administrative unit which provides a link between the urban government administration and the community. *Kebele* leaders were local party members, elected by the community, during the time of the Derg. They are now appointed by government as state employees. |
| *Kerray* | informal savings association for weddings, funerals, and religious festivals |
| *Kerray Abatoch* | the Elders of the *Kerray*, who meet to plan important community activities and to solve serious crime and local disputes |
| *Kiremt* | winter |
| *'kolo* | roasted barley or maize grain |
| **MCH** | mother and child health |
| *meda* | open fields |
| *Megabit* | March |
| *Meskerem* | September |
| *Miazia* | April |

6

| | | | |
|---|---|---|---|
| **MoA** | Ministry of Agriculture | *Tahissas* | December |
| *mogne bagenge* | a common illness whose treatment requires a surgical incision | **TBA** | traditional birth attendant |
| *Nehassey* | August | *tella* | beer brewed locally from barley or wheat |
| **NGO** | non-government organisation | **TGE** | Transitional Government of Ethiopia |
| **OPD** | out-patients' department | *Tikmt* | October |
| **Peasant Association (PA)** | the link between community and development or local government administration, with an organisational structure down to village level | *Tirr* | January |
| | | **TPLF** | Tigranian People's Liberation Front which, together with Eritrean forces, overthrew Mengistu's regime in 1991 |
| **PNC** | postnatal care | *tsebel* | treatment at holy waters |
| **PRA** | participatory research and action methodology which has its origins in 'Participatory Rural Appraisal' | **TTI** | Teacher Training Institute |
| | | **TTBA** | trained TBA |
| **PTA** | Parent Teacher Association | **VCH** | Voluntary Council for the Handicapped |
| **RTI** | respiratory-tract infection | *Weziro (W/ro)* | the term used for 'Mrs' |
| *samba* | lungs | **WFP** | World Food Programme |
| **SCF** | Save the Children Fund | **WIBS** | Woreda Integrated Basic Services, a UNICEF-funded programme including education, health, and water and sanitation services |
| *Sene* | June | | |
| *shamma* | a white hand-woven shawl worn by most women | | |
| *shurro* | a sauce made with finely ground chickpeas | *wogeisha* | traditional physiotherapists who are particularly used for setting bones after a fracture |
| **STD** | sexually transmitted disease | *Woreda* | urban administration |
| **streetism** | the trade practised by young female sex workers | *Yekati* | February |
| *suk* | small corner store | *zabanya* | a guard or night watchman |

# Executive summary

This report presents the findings and recommendations arising from a research and advocacy project initiated by Oxfam GB. The field study ('the micro research') took place in Ethiopia in the three months January to March 1999; the analysis of political and economic factors ('the macro research') was conducted in November/December 1999. The four study sites were selected to represent the diversity of traditions and culture, and livelihood structures, in Ethiopia. They included Cherkos, a slum area in the city of Addis Ababa; Delanta, the highlands of North Wollo (Amhara); the highlands in Eastern Hararge (Oromo); and the lowlands of Jijiga, Somali Region. Four detailed site reports were produced, closely reflecting the experience and views of the participants, and their perceptions of how the provision of social services, and their access to it, had changed over the past few years. Edited summaries of findings in four sites are given in individual case studies as appendices to this report. (There were five case studies in all; the first site selected in Jijiga had to be abandoned after two days, but sufficient information was gathered to merit a short case study, not reproduced here.)

A total of about 500 men, women, girls, and boys participated in the research. The research team comprised nine men and women, and more than 50 people were involved in co-ordinating and implementing the research. In single-sex focus groups of youths and adults, participatory research tools were used, including mapping, poverty ranking, seasonal calendars, and matrix ranking to explore health-seeking behaviour and the quality of health and education services, and Venn diagrams. The team was especially impressed with the information gathered from youth groups – with their level of knowledge, awareness, and openness. They made valuable recommendations for improving access to and quality of education and health services. In each site, individuals (70 per cent of them women) from 35 households were interviewed, having been identified during the mapping and poverty ranking as representatives of a range of groups: the worst-off, those of medium rank, and the

better-off. Providers of health and education services, both professional and traditional, were also interviewed.

The field study demonstrates the definitive interconnections between livelihoods, income, food security, and access to health and education services. It mirrors and compares the realities and problems faced by service users with those confronting service providers. It is intended to be useful to those planning and programming projects at local level, and to inform policy and planning at regional and federal government levels, and campaigns at national and international levels for the relief of unpayable debt and increased investment in human development – the planning of which should take into account the views of the poorest women, men, and youth.

## Main issues emerging from the four sites

- Populations are increasing; resources are static or diminishing.
- All households have become poorer because of drought, lost harvests, and dying livestock, and in the Addis Ababa site because of a huge loss of jobs among members of the armed forces.
- Increased poverty and loss of livelihood base (the male head of household's main source of income) have increased the workload on women in particular, and on girls and boys.
- There are few productive alternative sources of income, apart from selling firewood and petty trading.
- With the exception of Metta, traditional institutions, the church, and traditional practices are widely prevalent in the absence, or minimal presence, of external government or donor organisations.
- Women, their experience and concerns, are under-represented in all forums.
- In all sites, external donor presence was minimal, and some donors had stopped funding immunisation services, for example, without ensuring a replacement source of funds.

- In Jijiga, the site was devoid of any donor or government presence, no children went to school, and most of the adults were illiterate and felt completely disempowered.

The research identified numerous barriers to people's access to good-quality primary education and professional health-care services.

## Supply-side barriers

- There are insufficient schools and health centres to cater for the potential demand.
- Existing facilities are under-funded, ill-equipped, and lacking in basic requirements: books, furniture, water and sanitation in schools; equipment and medication in health facilities.
- Staffing in existing facilities is inadequate, and the health and education services are short of qualified personnel.
- Services are based too far from the rural population; the majority of users are urban.
- Outreach services, and health and reproductive-health education services, are under-funded and under-staffed.
- There is evidence of schools providing some education on environmental health and reproductive health.
- Traditional birth attendants (TBAs) in the sites visited have no access to training or medical kits.
- Herbalists (many of them men) have no dialogue with medical professionals.
- Both TBAs and herbalists tend to be elderly by Ethiopian standards (aged 60+).
- Few people have access to the system of exemption from health-care fees, and many do not know about it or how it works.

## Demand-side barriers

- Most people are too poor to meet the costs of education, which include food, clothes, uniforms (in Addis), exercise books and pens, and soap; and the costs of health care: transportation, fees, medication, nutritious food, bribes to guards, and lodging.
- Children are too hungry to go to school; many are sick with diarrhoea and other malnutrition-related diseases, and have no clothes; others leave school when there is not enough cash to buy an exercise book.
- Adult illiteracy is high, and an understanding of the value of education among parents is said to be low. Illiteracy also affects access to health services and other government institutions.

- Most worst-off households (the majority in each site), especially women, go to traditional healers or holy waters first, and seek professional advice only when their problems are very serious.
- The proportion of men using curative services is marginally higher than the proportion of women using them; preventative services are mostly used by women.
- Health education and reproductive-health education do not reach men and young people.
- Rural women use outreach services if the services come to them, but they tend not to attend clinics that are too far away from their homes.
- Most women and girls give birth in the villages without a trained attendant: health centres/hospitals are too far away and too expensive.
- Sending children to school competes with the need for girls' domestic labour and girls' and boys' income-generating activities, including traditional roles in herding and agriculture.
- Boys are given preference over girls when families have to make choices about schooling, most markedly in the Muslim communities of Eastern Ethiopia.
- Girls lack support, and their lives are at risk from circumcision, female genital mutilation, early marriage and early pregnancy, and a heavy labour-intensive workload from an early age.

## The official policy context

The government's policies on health, education, population, HIV/AIDS, and women's status all contain elements that purport to respond to concerns expressed in villages and by first-level service providers. But the needs of the poorest households and the demands of service providers, especially in terms of health education, reproductive-health education, and environmental health, do not feature prominently in the policy documents and cannot be met by the currently low budgetary allocations for non-salary recurrent costs, and with existing staffing and logistics capacity. Investments in improving staff training and development, and a significant improvement in logistics and management capacity would have to be made by the government and the international donor community, in order to work towards achieving the human-development commitments made to the poorest.

The gap between policies and demand is matched by a gap between policy intentions and the ability of existing government structures to implement them under current resource constraints, both human and financial. The process of transition to a federal state with increased local government autonomy is suffering from a low level of local planning, management, and budgeting capacity. Ethiopia's capacity to raise financing for social-sector development cannot begin to cover the cost of expanding health and education services and consolidating existing ones, which are very depleted. Ethiopia is committed to covering 55 per cent of its total budget for health, and 73 per cent of the total education budget, from domestic resources; but with 65–85 per cent of the population living below the poverty line, the state's capacity to raise local taxes is limited. At the same time, Ethiopia is crippled by external debt, and the interest payable on it (debt constituted 159 per cent of GNP in 1997; and while 0.9 per cent of GDP was spent on health, 2.3 per cent was spent on repayment of interest in the period 1991-97).[1]

There are demonstrable links between the low status of women and increasing population growth, infant and under-five mortality, and children's poor health and education status. Maternal mortality rates in Ethiopia are among the highest in the world, and fertility rates are 6-7 children per woman. All social-sector policies emphasise the need to change attitudes towards women and to recognise their contribution to development; but laws inherited from the past inhibit the widespread distribution and use of family-planning methods, allow for marriage at 15, and prohibit abortion.

At least 70 per cent of women and 60 per cent of men are illiterate. Illiteracy is an impediment to participative democracy and local account-ability. As a result men, responsible for their communities through traditional structures, feel impotent to seek assistance or take action to improve the condition of their families. Women are under-represented in all decision-making forums. Oxfam's research does not indicate that there will be a significant improvement in the educational status of the next generation, particularly in rural areas. The worst-hit areas are agro-pastoralist communities such as Jijiga in Somali region, where an estimated 88 per cent of children are not in school. Unemploy-ment in urban centres and the insecurity of drought-affected rural livelihoods are resulting in increased poverty and hunger-related illnesses and deaths. Hunger and illiteracy are impediments to local initiative and action, despite the strongly expressed desire of women and men to work for real improvements in livelihoods and for the well-being of their families.

# Summary of recommendations

## Financing social-sector development

- To secure the confidence of donors and to increase accountability between government and grassroots communities, the government should design and implement a fully trans-parent standardised system of reporting income from donors, expenditures by region and sector, and recurrent and capital expenditures.
- Donors need to agree on the format and timing of budget reports, to avoid demanding different reporting procedures and time schedules.
- To release new resources for meeting health and education targets, the World Bank and IMF should demonstrate a stronger com-mitment to the HIPC initiative and write off or significantly reduce Ethiopia's debt stock.
- The World Bank, together with the govern-ment, should review the impact of the economic liberalisation policy on the reach of non-salary recurrent budgets, which are currently not succeeding in maintaining basic supplies, including essential drugs and textbooks, to the health and education sectors.
- OECD countries should increase the proportion of national income allocated to development aid. This will facilitate the release of increased financing for non-salary recur-rent budgets for health and education, in order to improve the quality of service delivery and meet donors' renewed commitment to achieving human-development targets by the year 2015.

## Management and accountability

- Implementation of policy and management of capital and recurrent budgets at all levels of regional government require training, support, and motivation of local government staff, with technical assistance provided by local and external consultants, as deemed necessary.

- Attention must be paid to gender equity in planning, managing, and allocating resources at all levels of government and social services.
- NGOs can be engaged (with official development assistance funding) to mobilise and train local government organisations and community-level institutions such as traditional representatives, respected women, and health and education committees (with an improved gender balance). Groups of women, men, and young people, representing different clan, religious, and age interests, should be encouraged to participate in shaping and monitoring the development of health and education services in their areas.
- To this end, adult literacy programmes for participative democratic involvement should be planned and budgeted for.

## Expansion and consolidation of services

- There is a need to balance resources according to regional demand, for expansion or consolidation of health and education services. Expansion without an increase in non-salary recurrent budget expenditure for essential supplies, equipment, staffing, and staff training will not result in increased service provision. Some new health centres in Delanta were reportedly unused, because of the lack of staff and supplies.
- Expansion in health-service provision can best be achieved by responding to demands to take health care to the poor with outreach service provision. The outreach should be accompanied by increased funding for health and reproductive-health education and investments in food-for-work, water, and sanitation programmes, and it should involve both health and education personnel.
- Expansion in education provision requires regional and rural/urban differentiation; while the government concentrates on extending schooling to the poorest rural areas, it should encourage private-sector investment, for those who can afford it, in urban centres.
- Government capital expenditure should focus on under-serviced sectors such as agro-pastoralist communities, for example in the Somali region, and recurrent expenditure should concentrate on provisioning existing schools with much-needed basic materials and equipment.

## Reproductive health

- Reproductive-health education must be prioritised in view of the high fertility rate; the prevalence of female genital mutilation, high-risk births, and early marriages; a growing incidence of HIV/AIDS; and a high reported incidence of sexually transmitted diseases, which tend to treated only (and then only partially) by men.
- A rapidly growing population will constantly undermine the government's efforts to extend social-service provision. Population growth needs to be tackled with a carefully considered programme, and treated as an issue of human rights and development.
- Family planning should be legalised, and communications media and local-level organisations should be involved in campaigns to raise public awareness. High fertility rates and high rates of maternal and infant mortality need to be significantly reduced.
- There needs to be interaction between the education and health services in tackling reproductive-health problems, increasing access to clean water, and improving sanitation, as well as highlighting the risks of harmful traditional practices and HIV/AIDS. Non-government organisations (NGOs) can play a strong supportive role with external funding.

## Traditional medicine

- The government should invest in research into traditional practice, with a view to regulating bad practice and integrating valuable skills and resources into outreach services and service provision in health centres.
- The government should reconsider the benefits of training traditional birth attendants and integrating them into the formal health-care system, to provide a service at village level and refer high-risk cases to the local health centre in good time.

## Drugs

- The government should draw up a standard list of essential drugs and equipment, taking into account the problems of reproductive health raised by many participants. Issues of reproductive health feature more prominently in Oxfam's research than in the official health statistics reviewed, because most interventions are managed in the traditional health sector, outside the government health service. Stocking health posts with adequate supplies of family-planning methods will require planning and funding.

- Ethiopia needs an efficient system for the procurement and distribution of drugs (recommended in the official health policy), which would also regulate the drugs supplied via bilateral and multilateral agencies.
- Taxes on drugs should be reduced; essential drugs should be subsidised.
- Donors of Official Development Assistance (ODA) should provide additional non-salary recurrent financing to increase the stocks of drugs and family-planning methods on the official essential drugs list.

## Teachers

- Teachers must be trained and their skills upgraded, commensurate with the standard of the grades and the new curriculum.
- There should be a drive to increase the recruitment of women teachers, especially for rural locations. Special needs of women teachers should be investigated and acted upon.
- All teachers should have additional gender-awareness training to help them to understand the particular problems and constraints faced by girls and boys from urban and rural poor households. Oxfam's micro-research site reports would provide good background material for such training.
- A career and promotions structure for health and education personnel should be introduced, responding to the particular needs of those located in remote areas. Incentives to encourage applications for rural postings should be considered, together with investment in supervision and support for health and education staff.
- The translation and production of textbooks and teachers' guides for all subjects and grades need to be actively pursued and funded.

## Materials and equipment

- Investment is required in water supplies, sanitation services, equipment, and furniture for schools and health centres, including funds for the repair of dangerous structures.

## Secondary education

- Secondary education should not be sidelined. Provision for secondary schooling should be increased in rural areas, and made accessible to rural poor children. Special provision for girls from rural families should be made, to enable their safe attendance at secondary school in town, away from their families.

## Education for girls from Muslim families

- It is necessary to investigate appropriate and acceptable solutions to the problems of mixed schooling that Muslim parents envisage. Fathers in Jijiga were particularly concerned about sending their daughters to school with boys.

## Data collection

- Data collection should ensure that quantitative statistics, such as average class sizes and health centre/population ratios, are qualified by qualitative data, preferably collected from focus groups to reflect the reality of the situation on the ground.
- Oxfam's four micro-research site reports are a rich source of detailed qualitative and quantitative data, giving a voice to the poorest communities and providing information disaggregated according to gender and age from various ethnic and livelihood groups.

## Food security

- Relief and development agencies should work hand in hand with government and donors to ensure the supply of food alongside development initiatives, ensuring increased food-for-work programmes, relevant mother-and-child health services, and supplementary feeding programmes in schools.
- Investment in alternative urban and rural employment, to improve women's and men's purchasing power and economic and social stability, should be increased on a significant scale. Micro-credit programmes can fill the cracks, but will not hold the wall up for long.

# Introduction

## Purpose of the paper

The main purpose of this paper is to fulfil a commitment made to participants in Oxfam's programme of research on health and education in Ethiopia, the majority of whom represent the poorest women, men, girls, and boys, aged from 10 to 85, in urban and rural communities. Teachers, nurses, doctors, traditional healers and birth attendants, and regional government staff were also involved. They gave their time on the understanding that their experiences and recommendations would be transmitted to decision-makers in the Ethiopian government and international donor community. This process supports the aim of the World Bank/IMF and Ethiopian government to consult with civil society on the development of a Poverty Reduction Strategy Paper (PRSP) which, if endorsed, will qualify Ethiopia for the debt relief that it so urgently needs in order to finance development in the health and education sectors. The paper focuses on certain of the international human-development targets for 2015. These include the aims that every child should have access to primary education, and that real progress should be made towards gender equality, reductions in the mortality rates of mothers, infants, and children, and real improvements in access to reproductive-health services for all in the appropriate age groups.

The paper compares policy intentions concerning the provision of health and education services with the realities and problems faced by various groups of service users (differentiated by age and gender), and describes the problems faced by service providers and managers. The latter are trying to deliver health and education services in remote areas with minimal support and resources. The micro-research findings[2] demonstrate acute deprivation in accessing education and health services, and maintaining regular and timely use of them.

This paper demonstrates the definitive interconnections between livelihoods, income, food security, and access to health and education services; and the gender-linked disparities that characterise these factors. The planning process for the development programmes of the education and health sectors has been criticised by some for not involving the experience of non-government organisations (NGOs) and grass-roots communities. In this summary report, quantitative and qualitative indicators of villagers' problems in accessing health care and education are compared. Data collected on the allocation of funds between different services and between capital and recurrent expenditures are analysed, in the context of the problems and needs expressed by communities[3] and service providers. Problems of funding, management, and service delivery are also discussed. Links are made to wider policy and structural changes, and trends in factors related to poverty, food security, population growth, women's reproductive health, gender inequities, and livelihoods.

## Background to the research

Oxfam's Health and Education Research and Advocacy Project was prompted by concerns that many countries, including Ethiopia, are caught in a vicious cycle of deepening poverty and the emergence of virulent diseases. Economic growth and the distribution of benefits are impeded by national economic stagnation, fiscal crises, and the erosion of high-priority social services. There is now a broad consensus that the provision of basic social services can directly improve human-development indicators, including gender equity, and can enhance livelihood opportunities and facilitate growth with equity.

The fieldwork for the research in Ethiopia (the 'micro research') was carried out between January and April 1999, and the analysis of economic conditions (the 'macro research') was conducted in November/December of the same year. Four sites[4] were selected to reflect the diversity of urban, rural, and agro-pastoralist livelihoods and social structures in Ethiopia. They included Cherkos, a slum area in the city of Addis Ababa; Delanta Dawunt, in the drought-prone highlands of North Wollo (Amhara Region); Metta in the more diverse cash-crop economy of the Eastern Hararge highlands (Oromo Region); and the remote agro-pastoralist communities of Jijiga, Somali Region. A total of about 550 women, men, girls, and boys participated in single-sex focus-group discussions, using participatory research tools. Semi-structured interviews were held with selected householders (70 per cent of them women[5]). Interviews were also conducted with traditional, private, and government service providers and managers at the levels of village, *woreda* (urban administration), zone, and region; most of these were men.[6]

## Country context

Ethiopia is the third-poorest country in the world.[7] Its population had reached 58.2 million by 1997 and, with a growth rate of 3 per cent, is projected to grow to 90.9 million by 2015. About 85 per cent of the population live in the rural economy. The micro research indicates that 70–80 per cent of rural families live on incomes of $6.40 per month and spend 90–95 per cent of their incomes on food.

The population of the urban centres, where resources and skills are concentrated, is growing at an average annual rate of 1.9 per cent (1992-2000).[8] The country is characterised by high fertility rates (6–7 children per woman), shortage of arable land, recurrent drought, and climatic change affecting food and income from harvests and off-farm livelihoods, including those of women. Chronic malnutrition and widely prevailing income poverty, coupled with poor water sources (71 per cent have no access to safe water, and 81 per cent no access to sanitation facilities (1990–97)), contribute to a high incidence of communicable diseases which largely remain untreated. Poverty, disease, hunger, and the need for children's labour to sustain the household economy jeopardise the attainment of national development goals, including that of achieving universal primary education. As it is, 71 per cent of women and nearly 60 per cent of men are illiterate and suffer the humiliation, sadness, and frustration of not being able to provide adequate food, health care, and schooling for their children, the next generation.

Ethiopia's development has been disrupted by extreme events and trends in political and structural organisation and change. At the demise of the feudal regime of Emperor Haile Selassie in 1974, health and education services were underdeveloped, and about 95 per cent of the population were illiterate. The socialist regime of the Derg (1974–1991) brought the villagisation programme of the 1980s and the civil war with Eritrea and Tigray, which further overshadowed development progress and reduced the potential for attracting external aid.[9] The new Transitional Government of Ethiopia (TGE, 1991 to date) is committed to developing a market economy and a process of democratisation through the creation of a federal state, with many powers decentralised to the regions. The process suffers from a shortage of qualified and experienced women and men to plan, budget, manage, and administer the implementation of social-sector policy at all levels.

Since the introduction of an economic structural adjustment programme in 1992, there has been a significant increase in the country's debt stock. The UNDP estimates that external debt owed by Ethiopia increased by 93.6 per cent between 1985 and 1997 (from $US 5,205.7 million to $US 10,078.5 million). Ethiopia's debt-service spending is currently twice its budget for primary education. Overall official development assistance (ODA) fell from $1097 million in 1991 to $637 million in 1997 (before renewed conflict with Eritrea took place). This fact perhaps explains the large proportion of loan financing that is being used to fund the education sector, in the absence of sufficient grant aid from (for example) OECD countries. This reflects an overall trend in sub-Saharan Africa, where levels of aid have been falling steadily since 1994. In 1997 they dropped by $US 1.9 billion.[10]

Military expenditure was reduced between 1988 and 1996 from nearly 10 per cent of GDP to 1.8 per cent, and the army was reduced by almost 50 per cent by 1997 on 1985 numbers. Military activity on the border between Ethiopia and Eritrea became seriously intense in February 1999. This may have put a different light on these figures, and has changed donor attitudes to lump-sum budget-support funding, envisaged by the World Bank and the Ethiopian government for the new Social Sector Development Programmes, particularly in health, education, and food security.

# Structures for social-sector service delivery and public-sector financing

Four issues are central to the financing of development that is designed to benefit poor communities in Ethiopia:

- the ability of the national economy to generate sufficient wealth for taxation and public-sector funding;
- public funds allocated to the war with Eritrea;[11]
- the increasing debt burden;
- and the decline in official development assistance (ODA) from OECD countries, despite their commitments to human-development targets.

## Public-sector financing structures

An understanding of national income sources and federal and regional financing is necessary in order to assess Ethiopia's capacity to pay for health care and education. Fifteen regional states were established before the adoption of the Ethiopian constitution in 1994.[12] Addis Ababa and Dire Dawa are currently part of the federal state. All the other regions have regional state status.

Block budget allocation is made to the regions by federal government on the basis of a set of criteria, namely size of population (60 per cent), the level of social and economic infrastructural development of the region (25 per cent), and regional capacity to generate internal revenue (15 per cent). Regions with larger populations and those with a lower level of social and economic infrastructural development obtain a greater share in the government's total budget allocation. Additionally, the greater a region's capacity to generate local revenues, the greater the share allocated to it by federal government. The aim is to provide incentives to increase regional efforts at revenue generation. These resources are destined for allocation to priorities in education, health services, and rural infrastructure development. Budget allocations are made between the zones from the regional level. Where management capacity at zonal level is inadequate, the regional office provides sector-budget allocations to the zones. The zones redistribute the funds to the *woreda* offices.

While this has brought the administration of public expenditure under closer control by the regions, it poses a major challenge. All

components of the Oxfam research highlight the lack of planning, management, and budgeting capacity and experience in the regions. There are also indicators that, despite enormous need, poor management can lead to the under-utilisation of funds. Finally, women are seriously under-represented in the whole process of planning, budgeting, and prioritising the allocation of resources.

## Sources of public-sector funding

According to Proclamation No.33/1992, the regions are empowered to collect taxes on selected goods and services internally, whereas the federal government manages taxes and duties on foreign trade and the personal incomes of its employees and employees of international organisations. A third source of government revenue is tax from establishments jointly owned by regional and federal governments, large-scale mining, and forest royalties.

Recent fiscal performance shows that about 87 per cent of public funds is raised by federal government, and the remaining 13 per cent is collected by the regions. There are marked regional differences in tax-revenue generation capabilities. Income distribution in Ethiopia varies within and between regions. The region with lowest *per capita* income is Amhara, and that with the highest income is Harari.[13] Oromia, Somali, and rural areas of Addis Ababa have better income levels, compared with Amhara region.[14] More than 90 per cent of the rural population earn less than $1.00 per day. This means that neither regional nor federal government has access to the significant taxable incomes that would be necessary for adequate public-sector financing.

In 1997, Ethiopia's total GNP was $US 6.5bn. The share of net official development assistance fell from 20.6 per cent of GNP (1991) to 10.1 per cent (1997). The most important sector for aid in 1996 was agriculture, forestry, and fisheries. Disbursements for health and human-resource development amounted to 5.7 per cent and 8.6 per cent of total aid respectively.[15] Aid to support the recurrent costs of health and education services is negligible. External assistance to the country's total recurrent-expenditure budget is 2.3 per cent of domestic sources, and it made up less than 1 per cent of most regional recurrent budgets.[16]

The Ethiopian economy performed reasonably well between 1991 and 1998, compared with the preceding twenty years. GDP in 1997 was $US 6.4bn, 55 per cent of which was generated from agriculture, 7 per cent from industry, and 38 per cent from services. The World Bank[17] reported an average annual value-added growth rate of 3 per cent in agriculture, 4.1 per cent in industry, and 6.9 per cent in services. The low starting base, good rainfall, and the increase in foreign input in 1991 contributed to the improvements in agricultural output figures. However, the value of the main cash crop, coffee, has been in decline since 1986, and several regions of Ethiopia experience recurrent drought. Economic-growth statistics have to be read in the context of rapid population growth (3 per cent), widespread low-income poverty, and hunger. About 48 per cent of children under the age of five are malnourished. The Ethiopian government is not in a position to provide the funding necessary to meet international human-development targets without a reduction in the debt burden and increased external assistance that is not tied to long-term loan agreements.

# Poverty in Ethiopia

## Indicators of poverty

In Ethiopia, the major barriers to development and the main indicators of poverty include the following:

- the low status and under-representation of women;
- the fact that coping strategies have become main sources of livelihoods;
- the low educational status of adults and children;
- the increased burden of labour on women and children, who must work to earn income for daily food;
- widespread indications of malnutrition and high mortality rates among infants and children;
- miscarriage and anaemia among pregnant girls and women, and high maternal mortality rates;
- widespread dependence on traditional structures and practices for governance, healing, and childbirth;
- the persistence of harmful traditional practices such as Female Genital Mutilation (FGM), uvelectomy, tonsillectomy, all interventions involving children, and the use of blades or other sharp instruments.

## 'Worst-off' households, as described by urban and rural communities

Women and men in all sites stated that everyone was getting poorer, even those who were better off before the drought. The main source of household income (men's) had been eroded. Household food security had diminished to unsustainable levels, and the dependence on women's low-income petty trading had increased. Between 70 and 85 per cent of households in each community were classified as 'worst off'.

'Worst-off' households are those with a family of 10 or more, or with at least three small children. These households cannot feed, clothe, or wash[18] their children, nor send them all to school or treat them effectively when they are sick. They are households where the husband has died, or which have no reliable (male) employment and survive on intermittent daily labour (by men) or on the proceeds of women's petty trading. About 30 per cent of households were headed by women in Addis Ababa, Delanta Dawunt, and Jijiga; they ranked among the poorest of all. Worst-off households have no livestock and/or have no land at all. Households where either or both adults are too weak to work, or where there is a serious illness, are extremely poor. Children in these households contribute their labour to domestic, agricultural, and income-earning tasks. They cannot afford to use government education and health facilities. In all sites the poorest made fatalistic comments such as '*We pray to Allah*' or '*We lie on the bed and wait to die*' when they get sick, and many children are not in school because of their family's low income, or because of hunger and untreated diarrhoeal diseases.

The main 'shocks', apart from underlying climatic disasters, that seriously increase poverty are similar to all sites. They include the death or serious illness of the male head of household, the loss of a job or harvest, other serious illness, and death of livestock.

## Key development challenges affecting access to health care and education

### Low status of women

The National Policy on Ethiopian Women (1993) and the National Population Policy of Ethiopia (1993) highlight the low status of the majority of Ethiopian women as a serious development issue. The micro-level research found that women are seriously under-represented in local government, on school committees, and in traditional governing institutions; that they have less access than men to education and health services; and

17

that their reproductive-health status gives cause for extreme concern. They are highly likely to experience genital mutilation, early marriage and early pregnancy, high fertility rates, and life-threatening abortions. They receive almost no medical attention throughout their reproductive cycle (see the section on reproductive health in the next chapter). In all rural sites, men commented that women and children suffer more from poverty and hunger, and that women and girls suffer particularly because of their workloads, which include regularly carrying heavy burdens.

## Livelihoods and coping strategies

Ethiopia's Education and Training Policy (1994) seeks to provide 'relevant quality education to the rural population'. Rural livelihoods are no longer valued, nor are they perceived as sustainable. *Relevant* education is seen as that which provides skills required for livelihoods outside the agro-pastoral economy. Successive droughts and/or flooding have depleted livestock numbers, ruined harvests, and eroded women's and men's sources of income from crops, livestock products, food processing, and/or daily farm labour. Increased poverty in better-off households results in the loss of employment opportunities for women, men, and children in the poorest households. The fall in the value of the narcotic drug *'chat* (in Metta) has reduced incomes, threatened food security, and reduced access to credit for personal needs.

Global 2000, an internationally funded agricultural development programme, aims to provide seeds and fertilisers on credit to poor farmers, through a scheme implemented by the Ministry of Agriculture. The aim is to increase agricultural output. However, in drought-prone areas like North Wollo, farmers who have taken out credit for seeds and fertilisers and have produced no harvest are indebted to the programme. Participants told us they would be imprisoned for non-payment. Several men had therefore left the area in search of work in the lowlands to pay off the debts, while their wives and children remain hungry in the highlands. The challenge is to regenerate the rural economy with alternative sources of employment and income for both women and men.

Unemployment hit Cherkos, a military community in Addis Ababa, after the reduction of the armed forces in 1991. The loss of military-service incomes has also had a negative impact on informal-sector trading, services, and women's incomes. Unemployment in urban areas is also a major problem and begs the question: *education for what future?* Employment generation has to be tackled, alongside education reforms.

### Low incomes

Increasing incomes and purchasing power is central to improved access to education and to health and reproductive-health services. Reported monthly incomes in worst-off households[19] during bad months were as follows: in Addis Ababa 79 per cent of households earn less than $12.80; in Delanta 70 per cent of households earn less than $6.40; in Metta 70 per cent of households earn $6–$11; and in Jijiga 83 per cent of households earn less than $6.40. In Delanta, treatment for scabies costs $0.35, or two days' work for a woman collecting and selling cow dung.

Sources of income that were once secondary have become the main source, related largely to women's work such as petty trade. There are few alternatives for men or women: '*We are all struggling selling wood, dung, and wool. We are now tired, and the eucalyptus is also lost,*' reported men in Delanta. In Metta the men lie around and chew *'chat* all day, while women and children trade. In Jijiga everyone had fewer coping strategies than interviewees in the other sites.

Unemployment and low-income poverty are key issues to be addressed if access to health and education services is to be improved in Ethiopia. Women need income-earning possibilities that are less intensive in terms of labour and distance, and result in higher returns per hour worked. Men need alternatives to agriculture, especially in areas prone to recurrent droughts.

### Hunger and food shortages

Chronic malnutrition is a persistent problem. Farming families cannot produce enough to live on, and secondary sources of income are inadequate to purchase sufficient food. During the frequent droughts, livestock prices plummet, and grain prices increase. In Delanta, while grain prices increased, the sale value of livestock had dropped by 65 per cent. When livestock die or lose value, there is no safety-net left, and no food aid to maintain nutrition levels[20] until the next harvest.

### Children's labour

Girls and boys are significantly engaged in income earning and domestic work. In all sites it was found that girls' heavy domestic workloads free their mothers for trading. Children's labour is viewed as preparation for their future roles and is crucial to subsistence. Girls in Delanta said, *'If our fathers could get a harvest, we could go to school'*. In all rural sites, girls said that if there were grinding mills nearby, *'we children would not have to grind grain by hand'*. In Delanta boys and girls collect firewood on steep ravines to sell 15km away. Children cited accidents on the ravines as a main health problem. In Addis Ababa and Metta, children are engaged in street hawking and petty trading, girls alongside their mothers; this is a main reason for boys from the poorest families to stop attending school. Children in urban areas become vagrants: *'Our children sometimes beg or steal money for food'* (mothers, Addis Ababa). Girls in Addis Ababa and in Delanta Dawunt worked in the sex trade and in bars.

## Poverty, structural adjustment, and economic reform

The key features of the Transitional Government of Ethiopia's (TGE) policy reform are a shift to a market economy, agricultural-development-led industrialisation (ADLI) as the long-term development strategy, and the adoption of a macro-economic stabilisation and structural adjustment programme. More recently the Ethiopian government, together with the World Bank and IMF, is committed to the production of a Poverty Reduction Strategy Paper (PRSP) to replace the Policy Framework Paper. The PRSP has to be formulated with the close involvement of civil society.

The main elements of the macro-economic stabilisation and structural adjustment programme in Ethiopia are the following:

- tax-regime reform, mainly by broadening the tax base and reducing income taxes and taxes on foreign trade;
- controlling and prioritising government expenditure in favour of social and economic infrastructure;
- restructuring public enterprises for management autonomy and eventually privatising them;
- liberalising the factor and product markets and removing subsidies, so that resource allocation is led by market forces;
- devaluing the exchange rate and determining it by open auction;
- changing the investment climate to encourage private investment;
- liberalising the interest rate;
- a commitment to poverty alleviation and mitigating the social cost of economic reform through increased social-sector investments, mainly in education and health services.

Liberalisation, removal of subsidies, and tax reform reduce the reach of recurrent-costs budgets for health and education. The increased cost of drugs was directly attributed to liberalisation policies. Drugs are too expensive for the majority of the poor. The increasing cost of materials and equipment in schools, clinics, and hospitals also affects the impact that recurrent-costs budgets for health and education services can have on the quality of government services.

# Health status of the poorest communities

Women's life expectancy at birth in Ethiopia is 44.3 years, and men's is 42. Sixty-six per cent of the population are not expected to survive to the age of 60 (1997).[21] Maternal and infant malnutrition is a serious problem. Infant mortality occurred in 111 cases per 1000 live births, and under-five mortality in 175 per 1000 live births (1997). In the same year in the United Kingdom, infant and under-five mortality rates were 6/1000 and 7/1000 respectively. In Ethiopia there are four doctors and eight nurses per 100,000 people, with staffed services concentrated in urban areas. The micro research strongly indicates that most of the poor in urban and rural areas do not seek treatment at government health facilities, because they cannot afford to. Health centres are too far away, women do not have the necessary time or the money to attend them, staff attitudes to the poor are bad ('*They treat us like dogs*'), and there are no drugs available to treat diseases, once diagnosed. For many diseases women in particular prefer to visit holy waters or traditional healers. Men often choose to treat themselves at the local drug store.

## Main health problems

A survey by the Central Statistical Authority (CSA, 1999) shows serious levels of malnutrition in rural areas. In Oxfam's research sites, 45–60 per cent of participants reported eating two meals per day, mainly a handful of *kolo* (roasted grains). Health-service providers in all sites attributed the high incidence of diseases to poverty, hunger, and poor sanitation. Dirty contaminated water results in a high incidence of diarrhoeal diseases. '*Filth, lack of toilets, and the inability of the community and government to address these issues*' are contributory factors, according to TBAs in Addis Ababa, implying that the problem is one of poor organisation as well as lack of resources. The CSA survey (1999) found that 76 per cent of diseases are communicable, 20 per cent non-communicable (e.g. heart disease), and 4 per cent caused by accidents and injuries. The most common diseases found in the CSA survey were respiratory infections, diarrhoea, MCH illnesses, malaria, and HIV/AIDS. In all sites respiratory-tract infections are common, and tuberculosis clearly on the increase. Médecins sans Frontières in Jijiga estimates that 90 per cent of the population of Jijiga have been exposed to TB.

Participants in the micro research also reported a high prevalence of communicable diseases,[22] although HIV/AIDS and malaria were not commonly reported, except in Addis Ababa and Delanta[23] respectively. Health problems related to social behaviour, and those consequent on harmful traditional practices and the abuse of drugs or alcohol, were commonly mentioned by participants in all focus groups, and largely remain untreated and outside the sphere of modern medicine.

Men in Metta reported the side effects of '*chat* chewing, including gastritis, 'paralysis', impotence, and violent behaviour resulting in injury, sometimes death. The researchers noted other indicators of the psychological impact of poverty: signs of mental and emotional stress, including anxiety and fear among boys in Delanta, who said, '*We just want to live and to learn*' – not die of hunger. Delinquency among urban male youth and the abuse of alcohol and drugs lead to the harassment and abuse of girls, and traumatic injury as a result of violence or muggings.

In Metta and Jijiga, infibulation is practised (see the section on reproductive health below), causing girls and women life-long untreated health problems. Girls' early entry into the sex trade reportedly results in unwanted pregnancies and abortions. Miscarriage and anaemia, and heavy bleeding after delivery, were reported by respondents in all sites as 'main health problems' and attributed to malnutrition. A common complaint among women was severe abdominal pains, attributed to the regular demands on women to carry heavy loads.

Reproductive health is emphasised to highlight the fact that the government-sourced health-service statistics used by planners do not include reproductive-health problems among common health-related issues. All focus groups in all sites identified reproductive-health problems as being among their most common health problems. Issues of reproductive health must be made visible and expressed in mainstream health planning and budgets.

## Reproductive health

Women's reproductive health receives too little attention from government and donors, because it is allowed to remain 'invisible'. Legally girls can get married at 15; by law the use of family planning is restricted; and, while FGM is illegal, it is not mentioned in the health policy and is widely practised. *'We don't know one woman who has not been circumcised, nor one woman who has not had problems during delivery,'* said women interviewed in Metta. The National Population Policy states that laws must be changed and reinforced, and Information Education and Communication programmes must be applied if attitudes towards women are to be changed in reality.

In the Oxfam research rural sites, 0 per cent of women had been attended by a qualified medical practitioner during their last delivery (compared with 48 per cent of women in Addis Ababa).[24] Maternal mortality rates in Ethiopia are among the highest in the world, at 1400 per 100,000 live births (1990).[25] The delivery of Reproductive Health Education (RHE) is limited and very traditional; it includes family planning, immunisation, child health, and nutrition. In Jijiga 3 per cent of women had attended antenatal care (ANC) in their last pregnancy. In Delanta and Metta, 50–53 per cent had attended ANC on between one and three occasions. About 50 per cent and 70 per cent of these respectively had attended because the mobile clinic *had come to them.* The mobile-clinic programme in Delanta stopped when external donor funding came to an end. Health facilities reported an acute shortage of financial, logistic, and human resources to provide mobile ANC,[26] extended programmes for immunisation (EPI), and health education, including RHE services.

By using ANC and MCH clinics as the medium, only women (and in rural sites mostly better-off urban women) are reached. Men and youth are basically not reached. The only opportunity to contact them is through STD clinics, but most men reported that they prefer to treat STDs at drug stores or by visiting traditional healers, to protect their privacy and to avoid having to divulge their partners' names (a condition of receiving STD treatment in government services).

Reproductive-health interventions are mainly managed by untrained traditional practitioners in unhygienic circumstances, using rudimentary instruments, especially in rural sites. Male circumcision[27] affects 100 per cent of boys, who are generally circumcised as infants. The practice of female genital mutilation (FGM) is estimated to affect 85 per cent of Ethiopian girls and women.[28] Girls are circumcised in Delanta, Metta, and Jijiga as infants, at 5–7 years, and at 9–13 years old respectively. In most of Ethiopia, *sunna*[29] and 'excision'[30] are the most common practices. In Metta and Jijiga the more extreme form, infibulation,[31] is the custom. In eastern regions, impotence was found to be a common problem, attributed to *'chat* chewing and FGM. FGM is still practised in Addis Ababa, but the campaign of the National Committee on Traditional Practices in Ethiopia (NCTPE) has clearly changed attitudes and reduced its incidence. Although it is certain that the practice results in serious infections and heavy loss of blood, not one girl has been brought to the hospital in Metta after the intervention, because the practice is illegal. The doctor reported that very few come for delivery: *'FGM can cause obstructed birth, a ruptured bladder, and incontinence thereafter.'* In Delanta health staff reported that *'women and girls experiencing obstructed birth or other irregularities are most likely to die'.*

Girls were particularly concerned about FGM and early marriage, and they described problems faced by friends during delivery. Boys in Delanta and Metta expressed the need to address the issue of early marriage and the termination of girls' education. It is not unusual for girls from poor rural families to marry at the age of 10 and have their first pregnancy at 12. Abortion is illegal, and not socially acceptable in the rural sites, although practised in Addis Ababa and the rural towns. Illegal abortions in Addis Ababa have reportedly resulted in loss of life, and were the subject of great concern to all focus groups there. The victims are often young girls.

## HIV/AIDS[32] and sexually transmitted diseases

There were nearly 60,000 reported cases of AIDS in Ethiopia by 1998. However, the Ministry of Health estimates that only 15 per cent of total cases are reported, and that in fact

400,000 people are infected with AIDS and 2.5 million with HIV. Under-reporting is most likely due to the fact that most people do not have access to modern health facilities at all, and that many probably die of other diseases before being diagnosed. Of the total number of reported AIDS cases, 90 per cent of the sufferers are aged 20 to 49: the most productive sector of the population.

A survey of pregnant women showed an increase in infection from 13 to 21 per cent (1993 to 1997) in some urban areas.[33] In 87 per cent of cases, multiple-partner heterosexual contact is the main cause of infection. Prenatal transmission is also significant. A small number of cases are due to contaminated blood transfusion. Youth in all field-study sites voiced concerns about being *'at the mercy of health-centre staff and traditional practitioners using non-sterilised reusable needles and razor blades'*. The government's 1998 HIV/AIDS policy promotes the prevention of harmful traditional practices and illegal injections.

While all sites reported a high incidence of STDs and TB infection, the strongest awareness and highest reported incidence of HIV/AIDS was in Cherkos, Addis Ababa. In Delanta people know about the disease, since men returning from the lowlands are sometimes infected and die. In Metta, while men and boys were aware of the causes of AIDS, only one known case was reported. In Jijiga, while 20 per cent of TB patients in Jijiga hospital were infected,[34] there was a low level of knowledge about the disease in the villages.

STDs, gonorrhoea in particular, are very common, especially in Metta and Addis Ababa. The illness is typically described as a men's problem. Women are not recognising and treating the disease themselves. Sexual promiscuity in Muslim communities (Metta and Jijiga sites) is taboo to the point of denial and therefore needs to be addressed with informed and sensitive campaigning, particularly in the light of the spread of HIV/AIDS infection. RHE should address STDs as an issue affecting both men and women, promoting the right to knowledge and treatment for all, and safe sex practices.

# Health-sector policy and planning

## Historical perspective

Until the 1950s there was no official health policy in Ethiopia. Towards the end of Haile Selassie's regime, the World Health Organisation influenced a more substantive policy for health-service provision, and preventative care was emphasised alongside curative treatment. During the Derg regime in the 1970s and 1980s, health-policy priorities included disease prevention and control, with priority given to rural areas and the promotion of self-reliance and community involvement, and training and engaging Community Health Workers (CHWs) and Traditional Birth Attendants. The failure to invest in a comprehensive health system in the 1950s and 1960s, and the redirection of resources to the civil war in the 1970s and 1980s, have bequeathed to the TGE a system in need of substantial capital and recurrent funding, in the context of a greatly increased population.

The TGE's new health policy (published in 1993) is consistent with the aims of decentralisation and promoting 'the rights and powers of the people'. Emphasis continues to be laid on meeting the needs of the rural population. However, the policy does not fully reflect the gender-specificity of certain health problems, and the need to address the fact that access to services is not available on an equal basis to women and men, and that they have unequal opportunities to participate in decision-making.

## The Health Policy of the TGE (1993)

The policy document closely reflects international donor expectations of a developing-country policy. It has been further elaborated in various strategy documents, plans, and policy papers, including the twenty-year Health Sector Development Plan, plans for regional governments, HIV/AIDS policy, a policy on drugs, and a human-resources development policy.

The main elements of the government's Health Policy are the 'development of preventive and promotive health care' and the development of an equitable and acceptable standard of health service, accessible to all sectors of the population, within limited resources. Before the recent war with Eritrea, the TGE aimed to reach 80 per cent coverage by 2015. Support for the curative and rehabilitative components of health care, including mental health and provision of essential medicines, is also a priority. This is important, given the number of people who cannot afford to seek treatment: *'Many people die because they cannot afford health treatment.'*[35] The policy envisages user charges for those who can pay, and special assistance mechanisms for those who cannot (see 'Exemption system', below). The intersectoral aspects of health care are recognised to include population, food security, safe water, safe waste disposal, and environmental health. The policy envisages the participation of the private and non-government sectors.

Priority will also be given to Information, Education, and Communication (IEC) to promote public awareness of health-related issues. Health education is to include identifying and discouraging harmful traditional practices and discouraging the acquisition of harmful habits, including drugs abuse and irresponsible sexual behaviour. The National Population Policy also calls for IEC on women's status, family planning, and harmful traditional practices.

The policy is positive about the potential for integrating the beneficial aspects of traditional medicine into modern health-care practice. However, Oxfam's research shows that, while a few TBAs have access to training in some regions, there is no communication between health centres and most TBAs, herbalists, and religious healers ('holy waters' and Sheikhs). The majority of the people use traditional medicine in one form or another.

## Financing health care

The total planned budget allocated to health was expected to be Birr 5 billion over three years (1998-2001). In the Health Sector Development

Programme (HSDP1998), the TGE made a commitment to fund 55 per cent of this sum, in the expectation of external contributions equivalent to 43 per cent, and 2 per cent of the total raised from user fees: a total of 64 million Birr by 2001.[36] This figure assumed an increase of 09 per cent in user-fee revenues over the three-year period. During 1999, however, international donors suspended their funding in response to the war with Eritrea. Meeting health and education development targets will now take longer. However, during 2001 Ethiopia is due to come up to Decision Point on the HIPC debt-relief initiative. If Ethiopia succeeds in meeting all the conditions, new funds for health services may come available. Economic-policy researchers made the point that dependence on external aid for planning health-care delivery has been 'perilous', given the 'on/off' approach of the donor community to financing countries that are involved in conflict. A contentious issue to overcome with donors is the imperative need to maintain funding for social-sector development *despite* wars and conflict in African countries.

Public expenditure on health as a percentage of gross domestic product increased marginally from 1.3 per cent to 1.7 per cent of GDP between 1986 and 1995. On the other hand, the proportion of debt to GDP increased significantly from 51 per cent to 159 per cent (1988–1997). Ethiopia spends nearly three times more on repaying interest on external debt than on financing health services. However, the percentage share of recurrent budget allocations to health care increased from 1991, and the share to defence, until 1998/9, fell significantly.[38] The percentage allocation to health from the total capital budget also increased, from 2.3 per cent to 5 per cent over the same period. Real planned per capita expenditure on health care is still low, however, in the context of increasing running costs caused by economic liberalisation, devaluation, and rapid population growth.

The share of recurrent expenditure in the total health budget fell from 80 per cent in 1990/91 to 53 per cent in 1997/98.[39] This reflects

a recent emphasis on construction to increase the number of health facilities. Recurrent budgets are roughly allocated as follows:

- 37 per cent to Primary Health Care (PHC) facilities
- 1.9 per cent to training
- 6.5 per cent to anti-malaria programmes
- 17.2 per cent to administration
- 35.9 per cent to hospitals (used by not more than 15 per cent of the community).

These figures are representative of the distribution in all rural micro/macro research sites. In Addis Ababa, 35.3 per cent goes to PHC facilities, 3.9 per cent to training, 0 per cent to malaria programmes, 7.7 per cent to administration, and 53 per cent to hospitals.[40] These figures reveal a significant difference in administration costs between Addis Ababa and the rural regions, which might be worth analysing.

## Structure of the system

In theory, the new health system has four tiers of facilities, with a strict referral system between each level. At community level there should be one Health Post per 5000 people. Five Health Posts refer to a Primary Health Care Unit (one PHCU per 25,000 people). The next tier is the District Hospital, serving 100,000–250,000 people; beyond this is a Zonal Hospital for one million people. An emphasis on preventative services is envisaged at all levels of the health-care system. However, curative health care is also in great demand, as are outreach services. The field research showed that health-education and outreach services are seriously under-funded and lack an adequate number of qualified staff. The existing and planned structures do not match the needs of most rural and poor families, particularly women and children.

Statistics that are commonly used for planning, such as ratios of population per doctor and population per health centre,[41] provide a distorted picture of reality and can lead to

## Table 1: Percentage shares in government's recurrent budget[37]

|         | Health | Education | Defence    | Debt interest repayments |
|---------|--------|-----------|------------|--------------------------|
| 1984-90 | 3.6%   |           | 41.5%      | 6.9%                     |
| 1991-97 | 5.8%   | 16.7%     | 18.5%[38]  | 15.3%                    |

assumptions about the availability of functioning health care which imply adequately resourced and well-trained service delivery. In Delanta, only two out of five health stations are functioning. In Harari region, for example, there seems on paper to be enviable hospital coverage, but in reality the hospitals are barely operational. There are also wide disparities between regions in the provision of physical infrastructure. Predominantly agro-pastoralist regions like Somali region have very few health stations. Population/health-centre ratios are useful only if people actually use the facilities when they are sick. However, in each site participants reported that *'people cannot afford the fees, so they do not go'*. Women seek treatment only *'when it is really serious'*.

## Staffing

The Ethiopian National Health Strategy (1995) identified the following personnel-related problems: inappropriate staff mix, a shortage of front-line and middle-level professionals, and an urban bias in distribution of human resources. The WHO recommends a doctor/population ratio of 1/10,000 and a nurse/population ratio of 1/5000, but in Ethiopia these ratios are three or four times higher.[42] Given the urban bias in the numbers of skilled, qualified staff, the ratios in rural areas are even worse than the statistics suggest. The health policy prioritises measures to strengthen the human-resource base and management capacity in the health service. Instead of using CHWs[43] and TBAs, trained, front-line, community-based and middle-level health workers will be employed. Oxfam's research confirmed the need for more trained health personnel at all levels in the service, and more trained staff for health-education and outreach services.

Health-service staff complain of being demoralised, overworked, and underpaid, especially in remote locations. There is poor supervision and support, and a lack of the most essential drugs and basic equipment. The health centre in Delanta reported a shortage of everything, and no funds or medication for at least three months each year. There is evidence that staff are leaving state-funded services to work in the private sector, and that they prefer to remain in the larger urban centres. In recognition, the health policy includes plans to develop an attractive career structure, with appropriate remuneration and incentives, for all employees. There are no signs of this being put in place.

Management of the service is poor. Primary Health Care Units are managed at *woreda* level, but there is little attempt at accountability. There is a serious need to strengthen the planning and management capacity of the local government officials who are responsible for overseeing the implementation of the policy, and to strengthen lines of accountability between local government, the health services, and the community. In fact, few health-service providers had even seen the health policy or population policy.

## Traditional practice

In all sites everyone, and women in particular, tends to treat their own problems at home, and/or go to traditional healers. Many people consult the holy waters or the Sheikhs, who also do home visits. Of all sites, interviewees in Jijiga had less knowledge of traditional medicines and made less use of them. It was reported that traditional practitioners are close by and cheaper than formal services, and one does not have to wait for a consultation. The poor are treated with respect, and women in particular believe they will be cured. Young people, especially boys, were less enthusiastic, commenting that the herbalists were dirty and did not cure diseases. They want good diagnosis, supported by proper medical laboratories.

Traditional healers treat a wide range of illnesses. They perform interventions with sharp instruments, including delivery (which often needs an incision for FGM scars), tonsillectomy, uvelectomy, circumcision, and FGM. Traditional healers commonly treat men for impotence and STDs. TBAs treat girls and women for many gynaecological and pregnancy-associated problems.

The Health Policy envisages 'developing the most beneficial aspects of traditional medicine' through research and regulation. In Metta, however, government health workers were scathing about traditional healers. People are often treated in the villages and come to the Health Centres when it is too late: *'You can die waiting'*. The TGE does not envisage using TBAs.[44] In some areas TBAs still get training, but the impact is minimal, given the enormous demand. Since traditional practitioners are widely used anyway, the health system should regulate them, draw on their skills, train them, and integrate them into the referral system.

## Private practice and drug vendors

Very important to health provision are the drug vendors and pharmacists, concentrated in urban centres. In more densely populated regions there is on average one pharmacist to 600,000 people. In agro-pastoralist communities in areas like the Afar and Somali regions, there are fewer (1:1,000,000). The corner shop that sells painkillers, or drug stores, pharmacies, and private clinics are preferred and used for diagnosis and medication. Men are more likely to use this route than women are.

All participants complained that the poor are not given the same treatment as the better-off in government health facilities. In the private sector, they claimed, they are treated with respect. Women said the added advantage is that *'someone can go for the patient'*. While pharmacists have been instructed not to diagnose patients, they and the private clinics seem to be taking up the slack from the government services, and sometimes give treatment or drugs on credit or at reduced charges if the poor cannot afford treatment.

Private clinics want grants from the government to expand their practices. Both private clinics and drug stores want to be involved in any government-run training programme for health workers. Given that they are involved in treating reproductive-health problems, and STDs in particular, their involvement in RHE would be strongly advised.

However, for all practitioners outside the government health services there should be strict guidelines for practice and regulation. There are injectionists, healers, and circumcisers using non-sterilised blades and no painkillers, illegal abortionists, and many others who constitute a serious health hazard, particularly to women and children.

## Family planning and reproductive health

Ethiopia's National Population Policy (1993) describes the acute nature of reproductive-health problems. Fertility rates are high, and population is growing by 3 per cent per annum. Both the National Population Policy and the Policy on Ethiopian Women stress the need to improve the status of women: 'Vigorous steps have to be taken by government to remove all cultural and social impediment militating against their [women's] full enjoyment of fundamental human rights.'[45]

The policy states that without a reduction in population growth, the achievement of national development goals such as food security, universal primary education, increased access to health services, and extended employment opportunities will be seriously jeopardised. The school-age population, 12 million in 1984, is estimated to reach 42.5 million by 2020. Existing laws permit marriage at 15, and family laws currently in force restrict the right of women to regulate their fertility. 'Technically, all institutions providing family planning, including government, are doing so illegally.'[46] The prevalence of contraceptive use is estimated at 4 per cent nation wide.

The Health Policy (1993) pays special attention to 'the health needs of the family, particularly women and children', 'intensifying family planning for the optimal health of the mother, child and family', and 'encouraging paternal involvement in family health'. But real improvements require changes in the law regarding family planning, the permitted age for girls to marry, the availability of legal abortion, and an enforcement of the law prohibiting FGM. IEC programmes, drawing on knowledge and experience gained in Ethiopia and Somalia, should include media communications and collaboration with local government and village-level organisations, including women's and children's groups. Youth groups in all sites recommended education in sexual health for women and men, young and old.

## Drugs

The allocation of drugs per government-funded health unit has stagnated at the level that it had reached ten years ago. This is largely due to the rising cost of drugs. As part of the economic reform programme, drugs are taxed, and direct subsidies have been removed. As a result some hospitals attribute 80 per cent of running costs to the price of drugs.

One of the most commonly cited problems is the shortage of essential drugs. Patients from Addis Ababa to Jijiga, whether exempt from paying health fees or not, could not get treatment because the drugs were simply unavailable or were too expensive. The health policy (1993) clearly states the need to standardise the system, to prepare lists of the most essential drugs and equipment, and to develop an efficient system for procurement and distribution. Oxfam's research shows that there is still a lot of work to be done on this matter.

Drugs are also supplied through the National Drug Programme, via bilateral and multilateral agencies and NGOs. But the most frequently needed drugs are either not delivered or delivered in insufficient quantities and often close to the expiry date. Health workers reported their dilemma when treating 'free' patients. Health facilities run two drugs supply lines, one to treat non-fee paying patients (government supply) and the other to treat fee-paying patients. Often the drugs required for treatment, if they are available at all, are on the 'for sale' shelf, not on the 'to be dispensed free of charge' shelf. Drugs for sale are frequently supplied by a revolving drug fund, such as the one established in Jijiga by Médecins sans Frontières. However, most people visiting the health centres cannot pay for the drugs. Some health workers give drugs which should be paid for to poor patients, and risk facing the consequences afterwards. Patients in Addis Ababa believe that fee-paying patients get better drugs than they do. Poor patients most often simply go without treatment: *'We pray to Allah'*. In all sites, health workers and zone offices agreed that the majority of people cannot afford to pay for drugs.

## Exemption system

The majority of rural and poorest participants in Oxfam's research cannot afford to use the health service. Nor can many of these households obtain exemption papers to get health care free of charge. On the other hand, in Delanta the health centre cannot begin to cover its costs, because 75 per cent of patients (mostly urban poor people) claim exemption. It appears that rural households have less access to exemption papers. The Peasant Association (PA) said that only families with no livestock at all could qualify for exemption. Women are not as well informed about the system as men are: some women did not know, or even believe, that it exists. All participants who knew about the system said it was too complex: in some cases, by the time exemption was obtained, it was too late.

In the Jijiga site, no one was entitled to exemption, because there is no PA or *kebele* to process the applications. In Metta some women said that if the PA officials gave you exemption, you would be indebted to them, which deterred people from applying. In Addis Ababa the *kebele* was asking exemption applicants to pay Birr 5.00 towards a maternity unit funded by the World Bank, being built in the neighbouring *kebele*. Many people said it was not worth seeking treatment as a free patient, because there were no drugs for their illnesses.

More work needs to be done to improve the system of user fees and exemption, and in particular to address the differences between its operation in urban and rural centres. But it must be admitted that the health service lacks the capacity to cope with increasing numbers of free patients, and the drugs to treat them. Health-service providers confirmed that everywhere everyone is becoming poorer and cannot afford health care.

# Water and sanitation

The health policy of the Ethiopian government recommends 'intersectoral collaboration' in (among other things) 'accelerating the provision of safe and adequate water for rural and urban populations' and 'developing the safe disposal of human, and household waste'. An estimated 75 per cent of the population do not have access to safe water, and 81 per cent have no access to sanitation facilities.[47] In all sites the most common health problems were attributed to dirty water and poor sanitation. In the rural areas, the majority are *sharing water sources with wild animals and cattle*. In the urban areas, water contamination increases during the rains, and there are few facilities for the disposal of human waste.

In Addis Ababa there were open drains, overflowing public toilets, and streams of sewage overflowing down paths and roads and into houses. There are barely any pit latrines in the rural sites: people have to defecate in the open countryside. In Delanta there is one sanitation officer attached to the health centre, but no budget, transport, or team to facilitate his work. In Jijiga the women said that when there is no rain the dirty stagnant water does not get washed away, and they have no choice but to use that filthy water; everyone gets diarrhoea with blood in the stools. In all sites, boys and girls were especially concerned for improvements in water and sanitation services, including environmental-health education for their parents.

Collecting water is most often the task of women and girls. Boys from the poorest families also sometimes help in this task, and men in Jijiga and Delanta help during the dry season, when the water sources are farther away. Water costs money in Addis Ababa (but not in the rural sites), at 0.15 cents per 20 litres. In Metta there is piped water within 30 minutes' walk of each household, installed by the community with support from Oxfam. In Delanta, men and boys were digging a water source as part of a food-for-work programme, but they had not received food for the past four months. In Addis Ababa the *kebele* had applied to the World Bank Social Rehabilitation and Development Fund to improve sanitation, but since the *kebele* is too poor to make a 10 per cent contribution in cash, it is not eligible for this form of aid. There are NGOs, such as Oxfam, Save the Children, and the Ogaden Welfare Society, working on water-supply projects, but no sign of any serious and widespread national effort to improve access to safe water in any site.

# Food security

In 1994–95 Ethiopia was the second largest recipient of food aid in the world after Bangladesh. The Health Policy (1993) highlights the need for 'intersectoral collaboration', including the formulation and implementation of an 'appropriate food and nutrition policy'.

Most of Ethiopia's people suffer from chronic food shortages for much of the year, which give rise to famine situations as soon as a crop fails. *'Our women are malnourished and give birth to unhealthy children'*, reported men in Delanta. Infant-mortality rates in Ethiopia are 111 per 1000 live births (1997). Miscarriages and anaemia during pregnancy, and heavy bleeding after delivery, are common and are attributed to malnutrition. The National Population Policy links infant mortality to high fertility. The CSA (1999) estimates that 66.6 per cent of children suffer stunted growth, and 46.7 per cent are underweight.[48] In Jijiga men said, *'We are too weak to plough without food'*. Men die from hunger while carrying food aid home, or while carrying firewood to the market (Delanta). The lack of food security is responsible for general disillusionment among men, who express their sense of helplessness and failure at not being able to provide grain for their families, observing that *'our wives give birth to weak babies'* because of hunger. Many feel responsible for the suffering around them. Young people live in the shadow of hunger (*'If we eat food one day, the next day we don't'* ), and express their wish *'to live and to learn'*. Girls and women suffer more; women believe that *'girls can stay longer without food'*.

Low-income poverty, repeated droughts, and lost harvests and livestock reduce household food security. In the worst-off households, 90–96 per cent of income is spent on food. As cheap food for their families, women buy *guaya*, a leguminous plant known to have toxic effects.[49] Many families were eating a handful of roasted grains twice a day, and 85–100 per cent of households reported 'difficulties in maintaining nutrition'. Women cannot afford to follow advice on child nutrition. In all sites teachers reported hungry children in school, and parents said: *'Due to hunger we could not send our children to school.'* There is no supplementary feeding in primary schools.

In all sites women and men (and even the youth, in Addis Ababa) expressed the need for more food-for-work programmes. Supplementary feeding should be made available through schools and mobile clinics. Heath-education workers need to be more aware of women's ability to purchase or produce recommended foods at various times of the year, and they should provide support and advice accordingly.

Aid to Ethiopia has experienced swings between relief and development phases. They attract different funding packages, are managed through different government institutions, and are assumed to have different objectives and mixes of professional expertise. Oxfam's research in Ethiopia demonstrates the need to integrate these skills and experience, in order to plan and implement parallel relief and development programmes.

# Education status of the poorest communities

## Educational attainment in the community

Illiteracy rates in Ethiopia are high. In Delanta 70 per cent of the community are illiterate; in Metta the figure is 78 per cent for women and 31 per cent for men, and the figures in Jijiga are 79 per cent of boys/men and 98 per cent of girls/women. While there are clear gender-linked disparities[50] in access to education, both sexes experience a high level of educational deprivation. Nearly 60 per cent of men in Ethiopia are illiterate. While enrolment is growing at a rate of 21 per cent per annum, primary net enrolment as a proportion of children of primary-school age remains around 35–38 per cent (1997). The proportion of female students is approximately 38 per cent, and girls' attendance appears to be in decline, especially in Muslim areas such as Harari, Dire Dawa, and Oromiya. School attendance in pastoralist communities like Jijiga is negligible.

For the development of citizenship and participatory planning and implementation, current educational levels and projections are in urgent need of attention, particularly in rural areas, in pastoralist and Muslim communities, and among girls. *'We always talk about problems after they happen and do not plan for them before … There is no one educated enough to lead us,'* complained men in Jijiga.

## Perceived value of education

Providers of education services and youth groups believe that parents' low appreciation of the value of education contributes to low rates of enrolment and persistency, and high drop-out rates. *'Large proportions of children, and about 50 per cent of girls, do not attend school because of poverty, repeated famine, early marriage and parents' unwillingness to send children to school',* according to a *woreda* education office in Delanta.

In Jijiga, where educational levels are the lowest, there was a high appreciation of the value of education: *'An uneducated person is blind.'* Literacy and education are associated with the ability to negotiate and engage with formal institutions: *'to tell the government about our problems'.*

Women in all sites had mixed views on educating girls. On the one hand, they need to go to school *'so they lead a better life than us and get equality'*; on the other hand, *'Why do you need education to build a house and grind grain?'* (Jijiga). It cannot be assumed that all women value education for girls. Women's world-view reflects their subordinate status and their dependence on girls' work. IEC materials promoting education for all need to take this into account. Youth groups value education highly and see it as a means of improving the community, escaping from poverty, and getting jobs to support their families. Girls see education as a means of improving their status as well.

Education is widely considered as a road to employment outside the agricultural community, even though *'those who have completed Grade 12 from our community could not get jobs or further education'* (men, Delanta). Rural children lack access to higher grades within primary school and to secondary school; 85 per cent of the population and 6.2 per cent of all secondary schools are located in rural areas.[51]

## School attendance and drop-out rates

In Addis Ababa[52] only a small proportion of children attend primary school at all. In the poorest households[53] 41 per cent of the children in the families in the study were not in school. Of these, 67 per cent were unable to afford schooling, and 22 per cent had failed a repeated year.

In Delanta, 60–65 per cent of children of primary-school age were not in school. In Metta an estimated 65 per cent of boys and 75 per cent of girls were not in school. In Jijiga only five boys from a village of 170 households were in school. The education bureau in Jijiga estimated that 88 per cent of children in the region as a whole were not in school. In all sites, proportionately more boys than girls are in school. Generally the drop-out rate for boys is higher than that for girls, simply because they are greater in number. Table 2 shows that large numbers of children drop out during and just after Grade 1.

**Table 2: Low persistence in elementary schools**

| Grade | Wokote, Delanta | Ali Roba, Metta | Jijiga (town) |
|---|---|---|---|
| 1 | 253 students | 100–120 students | 100–120 students |
| 6 | 14 students | | |
| 5+6 | | | 50 students |
| 4 | | 27 students | |

(Source: Site reports 2 –4, Oxfam Policy Dept. Micro Research, Health and Education, Ethiopia, 1999)

# Reasons for not going to school

## Cost

The most common reason for not attending or dropping out of school was lack of money: not for school fees but for food, clothing, exercise books, and soap; for warm clothes in Delanta, and for uniforms and better housing in Addis Ababa. In Addis Ababa more children attend fee-paying schools. Registration in government schools costs between Birr 1.00 and 10.00. Children drop out of school when they cannot buy a new exercise book. There is no school in Jijiga, so the community had no idea of costs.

## Distance

In Cherkos, Addis Ababa, government schools are too far away, and many children who cannot afford private-school fees are not in school. Walking distance to school and unsafe conditions on the way are serious barriers to access to elementary school. Girls in Addis Ababa and other urban centres suffer abuse and sexual harassment on the way to school.

## Urban bias

In Metta and Delanta, the village schools stopped at Grade 4 and 6 respectively. To complete primary education, children have to go to town. This is impossible for most, especially girls, because of the distance involved and the cost of accommodation and uniforms. Girls cannot stay with friends/relatives in town, especially those from Muslim families. In Delanta rural children were two years behind urban children. Those in upper grades in town say they are discriminated against by teachers and urban pupils, because they are from poor rural families.

## Loss of main livelihood base

Shocks such as a drop in the household's main source of food and income, the loss of a parent, especially a father, failure of a harvest, or unemployment result in renewed demands for girls' and boys' labour. Boys who drop out of school often do so in order to earn income for the family. In Metta, 38 per cent of children quit school because their families needed their labour. '*If our fathers could harvest a crop, we could go to school*', said girls in Delanta.

## Domestic labour/early marriage

Domestic labour and early pregnancy in all sites, early marriage (at the age of 10+) in rural sites,[54] and abortion in Addis Ababa are all reasons for girls not going to school or dropping out. Girls' poor performance in school is attributed to domestic work before and after school. If a girl is in school, FGM and the three months' recovery period interrupt her continued access to primary education. There are inadequate data on early marriage, early pregnancy, and abortions; more information and openness are needed to respond to these issues appropriately.

## Children's work

In Addis Ababa, 67 per cent of children in the household survey were engaged in daily labour activities. In Delanta, of those in school, boys miss one–two days a week and girls two–three days, in order to work. In bad months and peak agricultural-labour seasons, the demand for children's labour increases and takes precedence over school. Women and girls have to grind grain manually; there are no grinding mills within easy reach.

### Coping strategies

Girls work so that their brothers can attend school. Some families manage to send one child to school, most often a boy, or send children for fewer years.

## Problems of accessibility and quality of education

Children, especially girls, with heavy workloads and inadequate diets, cannot meet the academic standard set by the Ministry of Education and have to repeat years. Girls repeat more frequently than boys do. Girls' socialisation as the subordinate sex, according to teachers, makes them shy and affects their school performance: *'Girls are victims of custom and religion.'* Girls do not know what to do during menstruation, so they stay at home.

Many children are hungry and tired in school and lack concentration: *'Children cannot work on an empty stomach,'* commented a teacher in Addis Ababa. In the highlands children are too cold and do not have adequate clothing. Diarrhoeal diseases also often reduce attendance.

There are insufficient teaching and learning materials in existing schools. Children share one book between five or eight children; in Jijiga town there is one book for every ten children, or no books at all. In all the schools visited, there are insufficient chairs and desks. Children sit on the floor, on stones or tree poles.

Some parents and children complained that the teachers are not up to standard, others that children are beaten in school. Discipline is a major problem in Addis Ababa.

## Teachers' problems

Teachers report being demotivated by low salaries, the lack of incentives, and the absence of a proper career structure. In remote areas they experience problems with communications, housing, and health services. Women teachers have no access to reproductive-health care, give birth without assistance in the villages, and have inadequate child-care support. There are no secondary schools for teachers' children. To provide competent instruction, they need training, textbooks, teachers' guides, teaching equipment, and libraries. Teachers respond to local poverty by buying exercise books for the poorest children and providing rudimentary education on matters of environmental and sexual health, but there are no educational materials and little liaison with health workers.

The translation of textbooks and teachers' guides from Amharic into the regional languages was raised as a problem. Some higher-grade books, available in translation, are used in lower grades. It was reported that not only could the children not follow the text, but neither could some (under-qualified) teachers.

# Education-sector policy and planning

## Historical perspectives

Limited secular education was introduced into Ethiopia by Emperor Menelik about a century ago. Under Haile Selassie this was extended to respond to the needs of a modern bureaucracy. However, the vast majority of the poor did not benefit. Participants in our research in Delanta and Metta recounted how during Haile Selassie's time only the affluent, urban population had access to education. As a result, disparities between regions, between urban and rural communities, and between males and females became fixed.

The Derg regime is associated with the expansion of basic education and an adult literacy programme which emphasised access to rural communities, highlighting the need for women and girls to participate. The TGE argues that the use of Amharic in primary education, in regions where it is not the mother tongue, hampered the spread of education. Moreover, policy objectives were compromised by the drain on resources occasioned by the war effort. The percentage allocation of total government budget to education fell by more than half between 1974 and 1988/89.

In Jijiga no Ethiopian government had built any school in the rural areas near the research site. There has only ever been Koranic schooling in Arabic, largely attended by boys. It is only now, as ecosystems fail, that the community begins to see the value of education for the development of alternative livelihoods. In Addis Ababa the introduction of school uniforms about two years ago has made education prohibitively expensive: participants say that it is more difficult now than ever before to afford schooling for their children.

## Education policy and planning

The National Population Policy sends a clear message: by the year 2020, the school-age population will have grown from 12 million in 1984 to 42.5 million at current population-growth rates. In 1997 only 35.2 per cent of all children of primary-school age were enrolled.[55] In the same year it was recorded that only 45 per cent of primary-school enrolees reached Grade 5.[56] The Education and Training Policy (TGE, 1994, p.3) states: 'The gross participation rate of primary education is below 22% of the relevant age cohort. Of these a large number discontinue and relapse into illiteracy.' The figures show a faster increase in enrolment than in construction of schools (4 per cent expansion rate), confirming the burden on existing facilities.

The cornerstones of Ethiopia's policy on education are *expansion, quality, relevance, accessibility*, and *equity*. Ethiopia is committed to achieving a gross enrolment ratio of 50 per cent by 2002 and primary education for all by 2015. The war with Eritrea has compromised Ethiopia's ability to fund these commitments, and the targets will need to be revised.

The planned targets of the Education Sector Development Programme (ESDP) are as follows:

- Expansion of enrolment from 3.1 to 7 million children (from 30 per cent to 50 per cent).
- An increase in the proportion of girls attending school, from 38 per cent to 45 per cent of total primary enrolment.
- Provision of one textbook per student in each core subject.
- Revision of curricula to make education more relevant and gender-sensitive.
- Improvement of planning and management capacity.
- Improvement in school facilities and quality of teachers to reduce wastage, dropouts, and repetitions to a more acceptable level.
- Increase in public funds to education from 13.7 per cent to 19 per cent of total government budget.
- Increased efforts to expand private-sector participation and introduce cost-sharing at the higher levels, Grade 11 and above.

## Financing the Education Sector Development Programme

Education is financed through public funds, external grants, and soft loans. Spending is divided into recurrent and capital expenditures. Government does not manage NGO and community contributions to education.

The total budget for the ESDP (1996/7 – 2001/2) is US$1799.2 million, with a 73 per cent contribution from the Ethiopian government[57] (van Diesen and Walker, p.23); of this, 16 per cent was pledged by donors. The resource gap was estimated at 11 per cent. Over the plan period, about 60 per cent of spending was earmarked for primary education, 11 per cent for secondary education, and 11 per cent for tertiary. The remainder would be allocated to capacity building, administration, adult education, and vocational training. However, on the outbreak of war with Eritrea some donors withdrew their financing commitment.

### Capital and recurrent budgets[58]

On average, 70 per cent of the total education budget is earmarked for recurrent expenses, and 30 per cent for capital expenditure.[59] About 90 per cent of the recurrent budget is consumed by salaries, and 10 per cent is attributed to non-salary costs.[60] In 1995/96 and 1996/97 the regions used about 85 per cent of the recurrent budget, i.e. the funds earmarked for recurrent costs other than salaries were barely used. Non-salary recurrent expenditure per student is on the decline.

Of the total sum of Birr 441.86 million allocated for capital expenditure, only 31.8 per cent was actually spent in 1995/96. This rose to 54.6 per cent[61] in 1996/97. This under-spending of capital and recurrent budgets reinforces the need for management support at all levels of regional governance. The micro research highlighted a very large number of capital and recurrent items needed.

### Allocations between primary and secondary education

Each year the primary schools sub-sector receives the bulk of the education budget. In 1994/5 and 1995/6, primary education received 60–63 per cent of the total budget, while secondary schooling received 10 per cent. In 1996/7 there was a slight change, with 53 per cent allocated to primary education and 12.4 per cent to secondary. The bulk of the modern-sector workforce is the product of secondary education.

In 1997 only 24.8 per cent of children of secondary-school age enrolled for secondary education, the majority from urban centres. Only 6.2 per cent of secondary schools are located in rural areas. Children in villages have virtually no access to secondary schooling, because of the costs and the distance from their homes. Effectively the few rural children who manage to complete primary education are denied the opportunity of secondary schooling. Girls have even less access, since it is not acceptable for them to live with friends or relatives in the urban centres.

## Management and implementation structure

Planning and budgeting begin at the *woreda* level. The Woreda Education Office prepares a budget request for new schools to be built. The budget is presented to the *woreda* council by the *woreda* administration for approval. On approval, the plan is sent to the zone, together with an estimate from the *woreda* of how much revenue can be generated locally. The zone submits all *woreda* proposals to the zonal council, which passes it on to the regional office. The region consolidates all zonal plans for approval by the regional council. Schools, like health centres, get supplies but no budget. Regions more advanced in the decentralisation process, as in Amhara and Oromiya, provide lump-sum money to the zone, which then manages the budgets. Otherwise, as in Somali region, where local government structures are not fully in place, the regional office manages financial resources. Teachers in Somali region often do not receive salaries and do not stay in their jobs.

In practice both government and donors recognise that the realisation of ESDP objectives is seriously compromised by poor management and implementation capacity. The Education and Training Policy envisages 'the evolution of a decentralised, efficient and professionally co-ordinated participatory system' (1994, p.5). Governance in the regions is so far lacking in continuity and experience; the capacity for management and implementation of budgets is inadequate; and there is a high turnover of staff in local government. While funding for the physical expansion of the service is insufficient, demands for materials, equipment, and staffing for the existing service also continue to grow.

External assistance is already called upon to assist in drawing up education-sector policy and plans, and needs to provide stronger support during implementation.

## Expansion versus consolidation

The Education and Training Policy (1994) aims to achieve one primary school per Peasant Association (PA). In Somali region, 31 out of 200 primary schools are not operational, and one-third of zones have no secondary school. In North Wollo (Amhara), 96 PAs have no primary schools. In Addis Ababa, schools are not spaced out evenly, such that children in poor areas have no government school nearby. New schools are being built in all regions each year, but transforming them into institutions of learning with all the pre-requisite equipment, materials, and teaching staff poses grave problems of supply, as well as organisational and institutional challenges. In Eastern Hararge, while efforts and funds are concentrated on extending primary-education facilities deep into the rural areas, old and urban schools are deteriorating. In all regions, supervision of existing facilities is weak, on account of the lack of transport.

Statistics such as pupil/teacher ratios that are used to guide the planning process towards expansion or consolidation of services are not applicable in the Ethiopian context. Oxfam's research demonstrates that the use of average figures distorts the true picture, by including the large class sizes and high pupil/teacher ratios in Grades 1 and 2. These change dramatically from Grades 2–3 onwards, owing to significant drop-out rates. The evidence indicates that if primary-school persistence rates were to improve, average class sizes and pupil/teacher ratios would soar well above the current estimated 60–80[62] mark. In that scenario, the case for expanding the number of schools would be indisputable. However, the maintenance of teaching standards also demands budget allocations to support the process of consolidating and improving existing facilities.

## Quality of primary education

The provision of primary education is not simply a matter of filling a room with numbers of girls and boys. While there are insufficient numbers of schools to provide elementary schooling for all, existing schools are overcrowded and under-resourced. Oxfam's research shows that the following factors affect teachers' and children's motivation and compromise the creation of a good learning environment.

### Materials and equipment

The quality of primary-education delivery is compromised by the lack of textbooks, teaching materials, and teachers' guides, and by the lack of proper equipment and facilities such as furniture, drinking water, water, latrines, and sports facilities. The buildings are in poor repair and in some cases dangerous. Like health centres, schools do not control any budgets for running costs and the purchase of education materials. Stationery and other items are delivered occasionally. Schools do not have a supply of basic medicines for common ailments.

### Enrolment and a conducive learning environment

Teachers, parents, and students talked about an environment conducive to learning. Large class sizes (especially in Grades 1 and 2), the problem of maintaining discipline, the use of physical beatings,[63] and an environment of poverty, hunger, and dirt, of vagrancy, traffic, and bars (Addis Ababa), were all quoted as inhibiting the provision of quality education.

While enrolment and persistence rates are influenced by demands for child labour, early marriage, and the poverty-related factors described above, they are also related to the quality of the learning experience while in school. On the whole, girls and boys want to learn, and education is valued more than in the past. Gross enrolment has increased, from 26.2 per cent in 1994/5 to 45.9 per cent in 1998/9.[64] The overall drop-out rate can be as high as 50 per cent between Grades 1 and 3, and children – more girls than boys – fail repeats and have to leave school. There are many constraints on children living in poverty, and girls have to contend with additional constraints. The gender gap grew between 1994/5 and1998/9 from 11.3 per cent to 20.6 per cent.[65] The education system still cannot respond to the needs of poor children, and to girls' needs in particular. The lack of women involved in the education system, from planning to teaching, from school committees to local government, exacerbates the problems. Girls do not believe that schools, and male teachers in particular, understand their difficulties.

## Staffing

Primary schools and parents' committees complained of a shortage of teachers, particularly of teachers with appropriate qualifications. Students also complained about the quality of teaching. Graduates of Teacher Training Institutes (TTIs) should teach the primary cycle, Grades 1–4, and diploma graduates the second cycle, Grades 5–8. Oxfam's research shows a serious shortage of diploma graduates, which results in ill-equipped teachers teaching Grades 5–8. In Amhara region, TTI holders are teaching Grades 5–8, and 50 per cent of teachers in secondary education do not meet the standard requirements.

In Somali and Eastern Hararge, there are teachers practising who hold only the 11th or 12th Grade school-leaver's certificate. In Somali region, 67 per cent of teachers have had no professional training, and only 19 per cent of teachers are women. Overall, women teachers constitute 27.8 per cent of all primary-level teachers. The education policy provides for special attention to the participation of women in the recruitment, training, and assignment of teachers.

Teachers suffer from a lack of appropriate training, lack of supervision, late salary payments, and the absence of a proper career structure. The education policy recognises the need to provide teachers with training to up-grade their skills, and incentives for those in remote areas. Summer programmes to up-grade teachers' skills are under way, but the coverage is not extensive enough to make the required impact. Teachers complained that there were insufficient training opportunities, and that political cadres gained preferential access.

## Curriculum

The new curriculum for Grades 1–4 makes a significant departure in content and mode of delivery from past practices. Teachers in Addis Ababa were not happy with the demands on them to teach all subjects under the new system. There is a need to 'retool' TTI graduates for the new curriculum. In some regions (such as Somali), the new curriculum has not been implemented at all. The curriculum for Grade 1 is developed on the assumption that children have learned numbers and the alphabet in pre-school classes. However, very few children attend pre-school, so they start Grade 1 illiterate. Some of the drop-out rate is attributed to this learning gap.

The education policy recognises the right of 'nationalities to learn in their language', at the same time as learning a national language (Amharic) and an international language (English). The predominant regional language is therefore the medium of instruction in primary schools. It appears, however, that translated textbooks are not available for all levels. To compensate, teachers with TTI training (Grades 1–4) in Oromiya, for example, use higher-grade books in the lower grades, whereby neither teacher nor students are able to understand the contents.

The education and training policy makes a commitment to ensuring that the curriculum is developed up to international standards, 'giving due attention to concrete local conditions and gender issues'. Education should 'reorient society's attitude to the role and contribution of women in development'; this commitment is also iterated in the National Population Policy and in the Policy on Ethiopian Women, and should be accorded planned action, time, and funds.

# The private sector

Government is the main provider of education in Ethiopia. Non-government schooling makes up 4.5 per cent of the total, and 36 per cent of private facilities are in Addis Ababa. Since the government focus is on expanding primary education in rural, indigenous communities, the non-government sector is likely to expand in urban areas, and also to include provision for non-indigenous children, such as the Amhara in Oromiya. NGOs and the private sector did not participate in the planning of the ESDP but are now represented on the Joint Steering Committee of federal government, regional governments, and donors.

# Conclusions

## Governance and human resources

Ethiopia has experienced three distinctly different forms of governance within the past 50 years. War and political insecurity have drained the country of resources, including experienced and qualified health and education personnel. The TGE inherited an underdeveloped, under-resourced social-services sector. The TGE has initiated a transition into a federal state with increased regional government responsibility, but the lack of experienced, qualified local-government administrators and managers is proving a serious impediment to the development of appropriate plans and budgets, and the translation of social-sector policies into action.

## Financing social-sector development

The transition to a federal state with increased local government autonomy is suffering from a low level of local capacity in terms of planning, management, and budgeting. Staff turnover is high, which disrupts the continuity of supervision and monitoring of plans, projects, and budgets. Supervision of schools and health posts is weak in general, owing to a lack of logistical resources and geographical inaccessibility. There is a serious problem in implementing policy and expending budgets in some regions.

Ethiopia's capacity to raise financing for social-sector development, with or without the war, cannot begin to cover the cost of expanding health and education services and consolidating very run-down existing ones. Ethiopia is committed to covering 55 per cent of the total health budget, and 73 per cent of the total education budget, from domestic resources. With 65–85 per cent of the population (taking account of regional variations) living below the poverty line, the state's capacity to raise local taxes is limited. At the same time, Ethiopia's total debt has increased to 159 per cent of GNP (1997), and while 0.9 per cent of GDP was spent on health care, 2.3 per cent was spent on paying interest on external debt (1991–97).[66]

ODA to Ethiopia is in decline. It fell from 20.6 per cent of GNP to 10 per cent (1991–1997). Of the total aid receipts, disbursements for health amounted to 5.7 per cent, and human-resources development to 8.6 per cent. External assistance to Ethiopia's recurrent expenditure budget is 2.3 per cent of domestic resources and makes up less than 1 per cent of most regional recurrent budgets. External aid, particularly to fund health and education recurrent costs, is negligible, given the enormity of the task and the rapid rate of population growth.

## Demands on recurrent expenditure budgets

In the education sector, 70 per cent of the total budget is earmarked for recurrent expenses, and 30 per cent for capital expenditure. About 90 per cent of the recurrent budget is consumed by salaries, leaving little to cover the cost of teaching materials, textbooks, and equipment, and teacher training. Non-salary recurrent expenditure per student is in decline.

Health facilities are short of equipment, essential drugs, and the appropriate balance and number of trained staff. There are inadequate funds for outreach MCH, education programmes to promote health and reproductive health, and for staff supervision and support. Despite huge recurrent-costs requirements, the share of recurrent expenditure in the total health budget fell from 80 per cent to 53 per cent between 1990/1 and 1997/8, and a significant proportion of that was used for staff salaries. Ethiopia spends nearly three times more on debt-interest repayments than it spends on health services.

The official policies on health, education, population, AIDS, and women all contain elements responding to the concerns expressed at village and first-level service-provider levels. However, the poorest households and service providers demand more activity at village level in MCH, reproductive-health education, environmental health, and water and sanitation services. The loud call to deliver health care to the poor in rural areas is not echoed in the policy documents or in financing commitments and cannot be met at current low levels of recurrent-cost financing, and with existing staffing and logistics capacity.

Liberalisation, subsidy removal, and import-duty policies reduce the potential impact of already small recurrent-cost budgets, and affect the price of drugs, which 'no one can afford to buy'.

## Capital expenditure

Allocations to capital budgets for health-care services have increased to fund the drive to build more clinics, but there are not the staff, equipment, or drugs to make existing facilities functional. In addition, while existing clinics are oversubscribed, the majority of the rural poor do not use them. Building new clinics without a major increase in recurrent-costs budgets, increased availability of essential drugs, and a functioning system of exemption from user fees for the poorest may not be the most appropriate way of extending health-care provision to the majority of the population, particularly women and children.

# Health problems

Hunger, poor sanitation, and dirty water supplies mean that 76 per cent of diseases in Ethiopia are communicable. The incidence of STDs, particularly gonorrhoea, is high and is seen as largely a men's problem. HIV/AIDS and TB are both on the increase. Many of the most common health problems, reported by participants, are related to social behaviour. They include the consequences of harmful traditional practices, FGM, unattended births, and the abuse of drugs ('chat in Eastern Hararge) and alcohol. These conditions remain outside the formal health service, untreated and not included in the statistics that are generally used for planning health care.

The Oxfam field study also brought to light the widespread negative psychological impact of extreme poverty. This included a deep sense of responsibility among men for the poverty around them, and a sense of failure for not producing harvests. A lack of motivation and aspirations results in destructive behaviour among youth in Addis Ababa, widespread paralysing 'chat addiction among men in Metta, and a fear of dying of hunger among children in Delanta.

## Access to health care

The majority of the poor, regardless of sex and age, believe that better-off people from urban centres get better treatment than they do at health centres. The poor feel discriminated against. Most people do not seek treatment at the local clinic, because they cannot afford to; they cannot get exemption from user fees, and in some instances women did not know that an exemption system exists. There are frequently no drugs, or no drugs supplied free of charge, so the patient returns home untreated. All participants complain that waiting time is too long at the government health centres. This is significant, because the poor, especially women, attend the clinic only when their condition is extremely serious.

## Fees-exemption system

The system for granting exemption from user fees, which is managed by the PAs and *kebeles*, excludes all but a few. Those who have obtained an exemption paper do not think it worthwhile, because, once they are diagnosed, the health centres rarely have the drugs in stock to treat 'free' patients. In addition, the exemption paper does not cover the other costs of health care, such as transport to the health centre, bribing guards at the gate, and buying food and sometimes lodging while attending the health centre. Women in rural areas tend to know less about the system than men do. Communities living in areas with no first-level government structure such as a PA or *kebele* (Jijiga) have no access to the exemption system whatsoever.

## Population growth

Existing laws permit marriage at 15, but it is not unusual for rural girls to marry at 10 or 12 years, and to become pregnant soon afterwards. Current family laws restrict the right of women to regulate their fertility: 'technically, all institutions providing family planning, including government, are doing so illegally'.[67] Contraceptive prevalence is estimated at 4 per cent nation wide. Fertility rates are 6–7 births per woman, and population growth is 3 per cent per annum. Maternal mortality rates are among the highest in the world, at 1400 per 100,000 live births. Both the national population policy and the policy on Ethiopian women stress the need for radical changes in attitudes towards women, and for improvements in their status. The health policy stresses the importance of paternal involvement in family health. But without a fall in population growth, the achievement of national development goals such as food security, universal primary education, increased access to health services, and expanded employment opportunities will be seriously jeopardised. The school-age population, 12 million in 1984, is estimated to reach 42.5 million by 2020.

### Reproductive health

Inadequate attention is paid to improving reproductive health, which, if addressed, may fundamentally redress many development problems. Untrained local practitioners manage most reproductive-health interventions and 'cures', often using sharp instruments in unhygienic surroundings. Girls' reproductive-health problems are potentially life-threatening, beginning with FGM, early marriage and early pregnancy, and a heavy workload from an early age. Men self-treat STDs at drugs stores or herbalists, avoiding informing their partners, who remain untreated. Official statistics show an increasing trend in the incidence of HIV/AIDS. The real figure is likely to be significantly higher, since most people do not have access to government health centres, or may die of other diseases before HIV/AIDS is detected. Men and boys have no access to reproductive-health education.

### Staff problems

Employees in the government health service are overworked and underpaid. Supervision and support, especially in remote areas, is very poor. In Jijiga, staff have to walk several days to and from the town to collect their salaries. The health policy recognises that staff are demotivated and that attention must be paid to improving career structures, incentives, remuneration, and supervision. The research did not find any signs of improvement in these matters.

### Preventative versus curative strategies

The research sheds light on the need for preventative outreach services, which would include MCH and reproductive-health education. There is also a strong demand for accessible clean water and for improved sanitation. Youth in all rural areas demand education in environmental health for their parents. These are some of the intersectoral issues that the new health policy aims to address.

At the same time, a majority of the poor are suffering from persistent communicable illnesses, such as diarrhoea and sexually transmitted diseases, which go untreated. All focus groups stressed the need for increased access to affordable essential drugs.

### Water and sanitation

An estimated 75 per cent of the population do not have access to safe water, and 81 per cent have no access to sanitation facilities.[68] In all sites the most common health problems were attributed to dirty water and poor sanitation. In the rural areas the majority are 'sharing water sources with wild animals and cattle'. In the urban areas, water contamination increases during the rains, and there are few facilities for human-waste disposal. In Metta there is piped water within 30 minutes of each household, installed by the community with Oxfam support. Otherwise there was no sign of a serious effort to improve access to safe water in any site. In Delanta there is one sanitation officer attached to the health centre but no budget, transport, or team to facilitate his work.

Water and sanitation are among the intersectoral priorities specified in the health policy; however, apart from Metta, there is little serious work being done to provide clean water and sanitation, despite the extreme deprivation in all sites, and the willingness of communities to provide their labour time.

## Poverty

Oxfam's research has identified some key demand-side barriers to accessing basic health care and primary education; they are linked to low-income poverty and isolation. The low status and under-representation of women are perpetuated by the dependence on traditional, male-dominated institutions of governance and continued acceptance of harmful traditional practices. With climatic change and lost harvests, emergency coping strategies have become main sources of livelihoods, increasing the burden of labour on women and children to earn income for daily food supplies.

The low educational status of adults and children, combined with poor health and persistent hunger, perpetuates a sense of impotence and isolates remote communities further from government and international institutions charged with managing the resources and process of development.

Everyone is getting poorer, even those who were better off before the drought. Household food security has diminished to unsustainable levels. Between 70 and 85 per cent of households in each community were classified as 'worst off'.

## Livelihoods

In all sites the main source of income, in cash or kind, has been eroded by persistent droughts and climatic change. There are few alternative productive sources of income for women and men, apart from selling firewood and petty trading. These are mostly activities which diminish local natural resources, and which are labour-intensive, with low income returns. There were no signs of large-scale planned investment in rural or urban employment or alternative livelihoods for women and men.

## Child labour

The subsistence household in Ethiopia is dependent on children for income and labour, which is viewed as preparation for future gendered roles. Adulthood starts early, from 10–12 years in some cases, especially for girls in rural areas, who have domestic work, marital, and income-earning responsibilities. Boys in the poorest households in urban and rural areas leave school to help to support their families. Work such as collecting water and firewood, agriculture, and livestock tending in rural areas and petty trading and street hawking in urban centres are common activities for both girls and boys.

## Food security

Forty-eight per cent of children under the age of five are malnourished. Oxfam's research shows that 70–80 per cent of rural families earn less than $6.40 per month, for an average household of six members; 90–96 per cent of incomes is spent on food. At the time of the research, a meal was described as a handful of roasted grains (*kolo*), and many reported eating only twice a day. Some parents drink coffee in the morning and go without food.

One of the main reasons for not going to school and for poor performance in school is hunger. There are no supplementary feeding programmes in primary schools. Women in Metta whose children were undernourished could not afford to follow advice on nutrition given by the clinic. TBAs link the high incidence of miscarriage and anaemia among pregnant girls and women to malnutrition. Malnutrition is described as a key factor contributing to the difficulties experienced during childbirth, to post-delivery heavy bleeding, and to maternal mortality.

Low resistance to infection as a result of malnutrition has increased susceptibility to TB in Jijiga, and to the more serious consequences of diarrhoea diseases in all sites, especially among children. Male mortality in Delanta was linked to malnutrition, as well as malaria and HIV/AIDS, contracted in the lowlands. Men in Jijiga complained of being too weak to plough without food.

# Problems in the education sector

The lead-in from the planning phase of the new education policy to the implementation phase is too short. There is no time for consultation and amendments before implementation. Many service providers have not even seen the policy.

## Accessibility

The government is largely responsible for education, and participation by the private sector is only marginal. In recent years enrolment has been growing faster than the rate of expansion of schools, indicating a demand on the education service which is gradually outstripping supply. However, the drive to increase primary enrolment, in rural areas particularly, leads to 'forcing' children into Grade 1 (Delanta), with a sudden drop in enrolment in Grade 2 onwards. In urban centres there is a growing dearth of space in schools, and many run a shift system to accommodate the numbers. Yet in Addis Ababa, education authorities reported that still many children do not attend school. Although official statistics report average class sizes of 60–80, in reality the figure in Grade 1 is often more like 100–120, while the figures for Grades 3–8 are much smaller.

Despite an overall increase in enrolment, the gender gap is ever widening. Boys are given preference over girls, most markedly in the Muslim communities of Eastern Ethiopia, but there is a high drop-out rate for both sexes. The main causes are low-income poverty, poor performance, failure of repeat exams, and household demands on children's labour time. However many children do not attend school at all, because most households cannot cover the costs of education, in which they include food, clothes, exercise books and pens, soap, and in

Addis Ababa uniform and housing. Children are prevented from going to school by hunger and diarrhoea, or because they have no clothes. Others leave school when there is not enough cash to buy an exercise book.

## Quality of education

Existing schools are not able to provide quality education because they lack basic textbooks (one book between 6–10 children), teaching materials and furniture, and there is no clean water or sanitation. The quality of teachers is not up to the standard set by the Ministry of Education, especially at the higher levels. The attrition rate among teachers is reported to be high in rural primary schools, and everywhere in secondary schools, because of poor remuneration, the absence of a proper career structure, and the lack of facilities in rural areas. The proportion of female teachers in the total is quite low, about 28 per cent at the primary level, and much lower at the higher grades.

## Illiteracy

Illiteracy is an impediment to participative democracy and local accountability. In Jijiga men went to the police station to ask for a school, not even knowing about the existence of the education office. At least 70 per cent of women and 60 per cent of men are illiterate. Women are under-represented at all decision-making forums. Men, responsible for their communities through traditional structures, feel impotent to seek assistance or take action to improve conditions in the community. Oxfam's research does not indicate that there will be a significant difference in the next generation, particularly in rural areas. Rural communities lack information and opportunities to participate in their own development. Illiteracy is a serious impediment to local initiative and action, despite a very strong desire among women, men, and youth to work for real improvements in their livelihoods and well-being.

# Recommendations

While it is incumbent on the author to make recommendations, in the interests of participatory planning and action it is the responsibility of readers to investigate and question further and to draw their own conclusions. The following recommendations are drawn from the conclusions of the micro and macro research documents.[69] By definition the majority reflect the concerns, interests, and needs voiced by the participants, who represent a cross-section of the population of Ethiopia, differentiated by age, sex, ethnicity, religion, livelihood, and professional status.

## Financing social-sector development

Dependence on long-term, maintained levels of donor funding has become precarious. The government has invested significant amounts of time in drawing up policies which accommodate World Bank criteria and other bilateral and multilateral ODA requirements. However there is no guarantee that funds will be forthcoming or maintained.

- The Ethiopian government, and the regions, should agree to full transparency in the reporting of budget expenditure, to increase donor confidence and allow for accountability between government and grassroots communities.
- This would require reporting on expenditures between regions, between sectors, between recurrent and capital budgets, and between preventative and curative health-care programmes.
- Procedures need to be standardised on a one-for-all basis, so that federal government and regions do not need to use up scarce capacity by responding to each donor's particular reporting format and timeframes.

The World Bank/IMF have made the production of an interim *Poverty Reduction Strategy Paper* (IPRSP), developed with civil-society participation, a condition to reach Decision Point in the HIPC debt-relief initiative.

- The World Bank and IMF must move fast on HIPC2 if human-development targets are to be met. Ethiopia's debt needs to be reduced to a level whereby debt service constitutes less than 10 per cent of government revenue. If the government can show that further debt relief could help the country to attain the 2015 international development targets, especially improvements in health and education services, then further relief should be considered.
- OECD countries should increase the proportion of national income spent on aid to meet the agreed target of 0.7 per cent. Long-term aid must be pledged now, to fund the realisation of 2015 targets.
- ODA should be directed to increasing the non-salary recurrent-cost budgets for health and education in the regions. Emphasis should be laid on increasing outreach health services and the provision of basic supplies and services in schools, including textbooks and teaching materials, safe water, sanitation, and furniture. In addition, supervision and support for staff living in remote areas need to be managed and funded.

Economic liberalisation, subsidy withdrawal, and certain taxation policies reduce the impact of social-sector recurrent-cost budgets, essential for establishing and maintaining the quality of services.

- The government, together with the World Bank and the IMF, should review structural adjustment policies in the case of essential drugs, medical equipment, and school supplies, including exercise books and pens.
- Import duties on free gifts to social services, such as operating-theatre equipment, should be lifted.

## Expansion versus consolidation

Ethiopia's population is growing at 3 per cent per annum, and most services are too far away for the rural poor to access.

- There is a need to construct new education and health facilities.
- This should be balanced with the need to improve the quality of existing services and the ability to staff and supply new facilities adequately.
- The balance between capital and recurrent budget allocations needs to be reviewed against regional needs.

## Expanding health services

- In the health service, reaching more of the poorest may best be achieved through an efficient outreach service and investment in water, sanitation, reproductive-health education and food-for-work programmes, in addition to improving the functioning of the PHCU structure, recommended in the official health policy.
- Schools should be involved in health-education programmes, and teachers should be given the requisite training in nutrition and the promotion of environmental and reproductive health.
- Construction of new clinics should take place where the need has been specified by the community, and if sufficient staff and resources are available to activate a service.

## Expanding education services

- The education service requires more schools; the aim is to build one per Peasant Association. The need is greatest in remote rural areas, pastoralist communities, and urban areas served only by private schools.
- Many more TTI and diploma-level primary-school teachers are needed to staff existing and new schools.
- In order to attract women and men into the education service, a good package, including promotion opportunities, needs to be offered, especially for rural postings. A definitive career structure with appropriate remuneration needs to be designed and implemented.
- There should be an effort to recruit more women teachers by identifying and responding to their particular needs, especially in rural locations.
- Practising teachers need 'retooling' training to equip them to teach the new curriculum; they should also benefit from new deals for teachers.

## Planning, management, and implementation

### Regional government level

- A programme of technical support and training for local officials is required, in order to improve programme and budget management, and to increase the capacity to implement capital and non-salary recurrent-costs budgets in particular.
- The lines of accountability between all levels of regional government, the health services, and the community need to be strengthened.
- The reasons for high levels of staff turnover at all levels of regional government need to be addressed and incentives introduced to reduce attrition rates.
- Attention therein needs to be given to gender equity, and representation and participation of various ethnic and religious groups at all levels of planning, management, and implementation.
- Technical support to improve management and implementation capacity at regional, zonal, and *woreda* levels via bilateral ODA is required. In 1997 about 40 per cent of total bilateral ODA was allocated to services supplied by donors,[70] including technical assistance. Technical support at local-government level should include locally recruited consultants, to draw on and strengthen national human-resource capacity and experience.

### Community level

Grassroots organisations such as schools and health committees, traditional institutions like the Elders in Jijiga and the *Kerray Abatoch*[71] in Delanta, Peasant Associations and *kebeles* should build their capacity to participate in the planning, monitoring, and evaluation of health care and education delivery. This is a process which requires training, experience, logistics, technical assistance, funding, and time.

- Attention should be paid to diversity, defined in terms of sex, age, religion, and ethnicity, and the need for equity in representation, in identifying health and education priorities, and in communicating with local government officials.
- Women and men in community organisations need to strengthen their capacity to communicate their concerns to local and regional planners.

43

- Local and regional government should become more transparent and accessible.
- One of the most pressing challenges will be improving the status and role of women at all levels. This needs to be addressed through a well-informed and orchestrated IEC programme with appropriate staffing and funding, linked to programmes to support health and education, food security, employment, and water and sanitation.

## Data collection

Data such as health centre/population ratios and average class sizes do not provide a true picture of reality and can be misleading for planning and evaluation purposes.

- Data collected for planning, monitoring, and evaluation should incorporate both qualitative and quantitative evidence, sourced from consultations with a wide range of age, sex, ethnic, and religious groups.
- Available data on the status of girls and women are inadequate. Evidence is required on the incidence of FGM, abortion, early marriage, and early pregnancies, and attitudes of the women, men, girls, and boys involved as parents, partners, victims, or practitioners. This information would assist in producing IEC materials aimed at reducing physical and psychological stress on girls, and also young men, and increasing the proportion of girls who complete primary education.

## Health

According to the women, men, and youth, and the first-level service providers interviewed, 'bringing health to the poor' should be a priority, alongside increasing access to essential drugs.

- In line with health-policy objectives to focus on preventative and promotive health services, outreach programmes should be developed which would include education for reproductive health and environmental health, MCH, ANC, and EPI programmes.
- Outreach services should co-ordinate work with selected traditional practitioners, schools, churches, mosques, Peasant Associations, kebeles, and traditional community structures, including respected women.

- Outreach clinics should carry essential drugs for the treatment of the most common diseases. Complications and high-risk maternity cases should be referred to the health posts.
- Funding for research and development of IEC materials, training for health staff and managers, staffing, materials, drugs, transport, and fuel needs to be secured.
- Funding should be earmarked for specific campaigns such as Family Planning, STDs and HIV/AIDS prevention, and discouraging harmful traditional practices, particularly those involving incisions, such as circumcision, FGM, tonsillectomy, and uvelectomy.

### Reproductive health

Reproductive health should be accorded high priority, both as a matter of human rights and as a development issue.

- Real improvements require changes in the law regarding family planning, girls' age at marriage, and abortion, and an enforcement of the law prohibiting FGM.
- Rapid population growth must be curbed and safe births promoted, to reduce maternal and infant mortality rates, and to increase the possibility of achieving and maintaining the achievement of human-development targets.
- Youth groups recommended that all members of the community should have access to sexual-health education.
- Women's access to information and treatment needs to be increased, as does the proper treatment of STDs among men, who tend to visit the drug store or the herbalist.

Female genital mutilation, a practice endorsed by women themselves, inflicts a most brutal intervention on girls and condemns them to painful and high-risk births, particularly in Muslim communities, where infibulation is practised and large families are sought after.

- It is recommended that experience gained by the NCTPE in Ethiopia, AIDOS in Italy, and Womankind Worldwide in the UK is drawn upon to change attitudes and practice throughout Ethiopia.
- Bilateral donors and international NGOs should support this effort with financing under human rights and democracy budgets, if they cannot find justification under health budgets.

44

## Local government and community action

- Local government should facilitate interaction and co-operation between schools and clinics to promote gender equity in the exploration of health and reproductive-health issues.
- The whole community, regardless of age, sex, or religion, should be involved in initiatives to reduce fertility, promote safe sex practices, provide access to treatment for STDs, and discourage harmful traditional practices, while maintaining values important to the community.
- Government, international donors, and NGOs must provide the financial and human-resource support required to instigate and maintain the process.

## Traditional medicine

Traditional practitioners are both a potential human resource and a potential health hazard.

- A more informed and explicit policy is required on the issue of traditional practice in Ethiopia.
- Research should be conducted in order to create a list of standards, to define legal and illegal practices, and establish lines of communication between health centres, schools, and traditional practitioners.
- The training and monitoring of TBAs should be reinstated, and funding provided from non-loan sources.
- Such a programme should be integral to regional health-care provision, including co-ordination with the nearest health post.
- Herbalists' remedies should be the subject of research, including audits of beliefs and values, with a view to formalising and integrating certain remedies into modern treatments.
- These practices need research and regulation, if not made illegal by law and enforced. The activities of 'injectionists' who practise in some urban centres should be made illegal.

## 'Chat addiction

- Consumption and sale of the drug 'chat should be made illegal, as it is in other countries such as Tanzania.
- Total social and economic rehabilitation of Eastern Hararge is required, in order for men to acquire full productive potential and assume their responsibilities as fathers and husbands. Women are currently carrying the load, literally and economically.
- Crop diversity needs to be introduced more rigorously to reduce dependence on this crop, which *'sucks our blood'* and which incurs the risks of all mono-species cash cropping: when the price falls, access to food, school, and health care is reduced too.

## Drugs

Oxfam's research shows that most people are not treating common ailments, because they cannot obtain or afford the appropriate drugs.

- The health policy (1993) clearly states the need to standardise, prepare lists of the most essential drugs and equipment, and develop an efficient procurement and distribution system.
- Drugs supplied through the National Drug Programme via bilateral and multilateral agencies and NGOs should be regulated and comply with the standards and requirements established by the Ethiopian government.
- Additional financial support to the recurrent budget is required, to increase the supply of drugs through health posts and outreach services.

# Education

Low enrolment rates should be addressed as follows.

- Reducing hunger and diarrhoeal diseases will increase enrolment and persistence rates.
- Increasing women's and men's incomes will reduce demand on child labour.
- Reducing fertility rates and introducing labour-saving technologies will reduce the demand on girls' domestic labour time.
- Increasing the age of marriage and providing reproductive-health education can reduce the incidence of early pregnancy and abortions, which cause girls to drop out or not attend school at all.
- Organising schooling around the agricultural calendar and introducing shifts at certain times of the year will enable children to co-ordinate schooling with agricultural work.
- Campaigns should be organised to increase women's and men's awareness of the value of education.
- Schools should be involved in environmental-health and reproductive-health programmes.
- More women should be recruited to serve on school committees.

- The number of women teachers should be increased, to respond to the particular needs of girls.
- Discussions should be held with Muslim communities to develop strategies for educating girls and boys separately, and acceptable ways of educating them together, to increase girls' access to education.

### Human resources

Teachers require upgrading training commensurate with the standards of the grades and curriculum that they are teaching.

- The teacher-training curriculum should include preparation for life in remote and poor communities, with insights into differences between girls' and boys' experience of poverty.
- Teachers should also have elementary training in basic health education, reproductive-health issues, and water and sanitation matters, to facilitate their collaboration with community groups and the health centre.
- The Oxfam Policy Department Micro Research Site Reports Nos. 1 – 4 would provide useful background and training material, and also insights into participatory learning and action techniques.
- Resources should be directed at translating textbooks and teachers' guides into national languages for all primary-school subject areas, and teachers should be teaching with the appropriate texts and levels for each grade.
- Non-salary recurrent budgets need inputs to increase the availability of textbooks.
- Investment in providing teachers' desks and chairs and desks for children is required.
- The provision of clean water and basic sanitation needs community action and external funding.
- Provision of basic medical supplies and supplementary feeding would reduce the anxiety felt by teachers faced with sick, hungry, and tired children and would increase motivation to teach and to learn.

### Private sector

- Regional governments should provide incentives to the private sector by allocating land for expanding non-government education facilities in the towns and rural areas.

### Drop-outs

The absence of pre-school preparation is given as one reason for the high first-grade drop-out rate.

- Grade 1 should be treated as the first introduction to basic skills in reading, writing, and numeracy, and the curriculum should be adjusted accordingly.

### Secondary education

In the drive for primary education, secondary education is being left behind, with very poor coverage in rural areas. Low enrolment is also attributed to the fact that there are no opportunities for further education in rural areas.

- There needs to be one secondary school per *woreda*.
- Children from rural families, particularly girls, need to be integrated and accommodated.
- Funds for teacher training, school equipment, and supplies, including textbooks and teaching materials, are required.

### Non-indigenous children

- Federal and regional governments need to develop a policy framework to accommodate non-indigenous children, where the size of population warrants the establishment of separate schools.

## Food security

Aid to Ethiopia has experienced swings between relief and development phases. They attract different funding packages, are managed through different government institutions, and are assumed to have different objectives and mixes of professional expertise.

- Oxfam's research in Ethiopia demonstrates the need to integrate these skills and experience for the planning and programming of parallel relief and development programmes.
- Food-for-work programmes were requested in all sites.
- Supplementary feeding in primary schools would improve performance and may increase attendance.
- Women should be provided with appropriate nutrition advice, and/or supplementary feeding for infants. Alternative employment to increase women's purchasing power would be the longer-term solution.

Unemployment and low-income poverty are key issues to be addressed if access to food, health services, and education is to be improved. The rural areas visited, including their urban centres, are devoid of any serious attempts to introduce programmes for employment generation or rural industrialisation.

- Women need incoming-earning opportunities that are closer to their homes and less labour-intensive, and permit more value to be added to their work.
- Men need alternatives to agriculture, especially in areas prone to recurrent droughts.
- Micro-credit support for existing rural livelihoods should be accompanied by investment in alternative rural livelihoods for women and men, alongside literacy and numeracy programmes.

## Water and sanitation

- Widespread clean-water programmes are required; communities are ready to contribute their labour on a food-for-work basis, but in those cases food must be provided.
- Sanitation and pit-latrine programmes should be instigated, using relief-work experience and mobilising communities through schools and outreach health clinics.
- In urban centres the World Bank Social Rehabilitation and Development Fund programme should accept labour instead of cash, in order to extend financing for water and sanitation to the poorest urban communities. At current income levels, the need to provide cash contributions can mean that a child must leave school, food is reduced, or an illness is left untreated.

# Notes

1   Ministry for Economic Development and Co-operation (1999).

2   Oxfam Policy Department Micro Research: Health and Education Ethiopia: Site Report No. 1 Cherkos Addis Ababa;  Site Report No.2 Yegurassa and Andaje, Delanta Dawunt; Site Report No.3 Ali Roba, Metta; Site Report No.4 Belhare, Jijiga.

3   'Communities' includes women, men, girls, and boys.

4   Detailed site reports have been produced which closely reflect the experience and views of the participants.

5   A larger proportion of women than men, in the reproductive-age group, were interviewed, since the questionnaires had a strong focus on women's reproductive health.

6   For micro-research methodology, see Appendix 1.

7   UNDP *Human Development Report* 1999.

8   UNDP *Human Development Report* 1995.

9   *The Changing Face of Aid to Ethiopia*, Christian Aid 1999 p.6.

10  *The Reality of Aid 2000*, Earthscan Publications 2000.

11  This paper does not attempt or intend to analyse, comment on, or judge the Ethiopian government financing of the war with Eritrea. It was a coincidence that the war broke out in earnest during the micro-research phase. It was not within the remit of the research objectives to consider the issue of prioritising the allocation of financial resources in war-time.

12  Tigrai (Region 1), Afar (Region 2), Amhara (Region 3), Oromia (Region 4), Somali (Region 5), Benshangul Gumuz (Region 6), Southern Nations Nationalities and Peoples Region (a region formed by Regions numbered 7 to 11 during the transitional period before 1994), Gambella (Region 12), Harari (Region 13), Addis Ababa (Region 14) and Dire Dawa (Region 15).

13  This may be an indication of sales of 'chat, coffee, and contraband items.

14  A major consideration should be the level of price differentials among the regions. The purchasing power of the Birr differs from area to area.

15  *The Changing Face of Aid to Ethiopia*, Christian Aid 1999.

16  MOE planning and programming panel.

17  *World Development Report*, World Bank 1998/99.

18  Washing requires a change of clothes, and access to clean water and soap; under the current gendered division of labour it also requires women's time. Women are out trading to earn 1.00 – 3.00 Birr per day to feed families of six.

19  Average household size in worst-off households: six members.

20  This was the situation on the ground at the time of the micro research, January–March 1999. Food aid was subsequently distributed to North Wollo and (much later) to Somali region.

21  UNDP *Human Development Report*, 1999.

22  See Table 3 in Appendix 2.

23  Men working in the lowlands often return with malaria and die.

24  92 per cent of deliveries in Ethiopia are not attended by a medical or skilled attendant (UNFPA, 1999).

25  In the UK, maternal mortality is 9 cases per 100,000 live births, and in the USA 12 per 100,000.

26  ANC: Ante-Natal Care; EPI: Extended Programme of Immunisation; MCH: Mother and Child Health.

27  Male circumcision has never been referred to as genital mutilation. Some men's groups in Egypt are beginning to question the practice and raise awareness about potential reproductive health hazards for boys and men.

28  B. Spadacini and P. Nichols in *Gender and Development*, Vol 6 No 2 July 1998.

29  *Sunna*: the hood of the clitoris is removed.

30  *Excision*: the clitoris and all or part of the labia minora are removed.

31  Infibulation: removal of the clitoris, labia majora, and labia minora, and stitching with thorns, binding the legs until the wound heals, to leave a small hole for urine and menstrual flow.

32  This section heavily relies on MOH (Epidemiology and AIDS department): *AIDS in Ethiopia 2nd edition* Addis Ababa (1998).

33  See Table 4 in Appendix 2.

34    Reported by MSF Belgium, Jijiga.

35    Micro Research Health and Education, Ethiopia 1999: women in Delanta, echoing voices in all sites.

36    See Tables 5 and 6 in Appendix 2.

37    MEDAC 1999, Oxfam Policy Department Macro Research Health Sector report 1999 p. 38.

38    1999–2000 defence expenditures were not available at the time of writing.

39    See Table 7 in Appendix 2.

40    Macro research: Health and Education, Ethiopia 1999 pp.46-7.

41    See Tables 9 and 10 in Appendix 2.

42    See Table 9 in Appendix 2.

43    CHW: Community Health Worker – members of the community in the Derg's time.

44    TBA: Traditional birth attendant.

45    National Population Policy p.20 (1993).

46    Op cit. p.18.

47    UNDP *Human Development Report* 1999.

48    See Table 11 in Appendix 2 for regional differences in infant and under-5 mortality and life expectancy.

49    *Guaya* or vetch (*Lattiru sattirus*) is a drought-resistant leguminous plant, resembling the chick pea. It produces a neuro-toxic substance called aflatoxin, which affects the nervous system and can cause lameness. The disease associated with the consumption of *guaya* is called lattirism.

50    Female net enrolment as % of male ratio: primary 62%, secondary 55%, tertiary 24% (1997).

51    See Table 12 in Appendix 2 for rural–urban distribution of schools by region.

52    Zone 2 Education Office, Addis Ababa, January 1999.

53    Source: Oxfam Policy Department Micro Research: household survey (1999).

54    In some parts of Ethiopia, kidnapping young girls into marriage is also common, but this issue was not raised during this research.

55    See Table 13 in Appendix 2.

56    UNDP *Human Development Report* 1999.

57    Christian Aid: *The Changing Face of Aid to Ethiopia* (1999).

58    See Table 14 in Appendix 2.

59    There are regional variations: Amhara allocated 83% to the recurrent budget and 17% to the capital budget. Non-salary recurrent expenditures remain very low and affect the quality of education in the region.

60    MOE planning and programming panel 1994/5 – 1996/7.

61    Oxfam Policy Department Macro Research: Health and Education, Ethiopia (1999).

62    Oxfam Policy Department Micro Research: Health and Education, Ethiopia (1999).

63    Parents and children complained about beatings in Addis Ababa and Wollo.

64    In agro-pastoralist communities such as Somali region, enrolment is desperately low: 5.95% of boys and 3.74% of girls in 1998/9, an increase of 9.7% on 1997/8.

65    Oxfam Policy Dept. Macro Research: Health and Education, Ethiopia 1999 p.43.

66    MEDAC 1999.

67    Op cit. p.18

68    UNDP *Human Development Report* 1999.

69    There are four detailed micro-research site-reports; a summary of the micro research findings, a macro health report; and a macro education report.

70    Refers to all recipient countries (*The Reality of Aid* p. 4, Earthscan 2000).

71    Identified as one of the most important social institutions in Delanta. All households are represented and make contributions. The Elders (*Abatoch*) meet to organise large community events around religious festivals or marriages and deaths. They also act as a court and preside over disputes and crimes. The worst punishment is to be banished from the church.

72    PRA: Participatory Research and Action.

73    There were more translators, but not all were involved in the focus-group discussions when the PRA techniques were applied.

74    Including two separate locations in Jijiga.

75    In Addis *samba* (lung) is a nickname for HIV/AIDS. Participants explained that when people, especially young men, do not respond to TB treatment, it is assumed that they have AIDS.

76    Mogne Bagne: fever, chills, nausea, abdominal distension treated with an incision by herbalists.

77    A common problem treated by herbalists and perhaps associated with '*chat* consumption. Produces fever and rheumatic pains.

78    Land disputes between male relations and domestic violence against women and children – violence attributed to '*chat* consumption.

79    Performed by a traditional practitioner with a razor or sharp instrument.

80    Research sites in italics.

81    In Ethiopia as a whole, men's average life expectancy is 49.7 years and women's 52.4.

82    Research sites in italics.

49

# References and further reading

**Kello, Abdulhamid Bedri and Getachew Yoseph** (1999) Oxfam Policy Department Health Sector Ethiopia Macro Report

**Kello, Abdulhamid Bedri and Getachew Yoseph** (1999) Oxfam Policy Department Education Sector Ethiopia, Macro Report

**von Massow, F., A. Terefe, A. Bekele, S. Feyissa, T. Haile, A. Kidane Gebrehiwot, T. Koyra, A. Worku, and D. Zewdie** (1999) Oxfam Policy Department Micro Research: Health and Education Ethiopia, Site Report No. 1 Cherkos, Addis Ababa

**von Massow, F., A. Terefe, A. Bekele, S. Feyissa, T. Haile, A. Kidane Gebrehiwot, T. Koyra, A. Worku, and D. Zewdie** (1999) Oxfam Policy Department Micro Research: Health and Education Ethiopia, Site Report No. 2. Delanta Dawunt, North Wollo

**von Massow, F., A. Terefe, A. Bekele, S. Feyissa, T. Haile, A. Kidane Gebrehiwot, T. Koyra, A. Worku, and D. Zewdie** (1999) Oxfam Policy Department Micro Research: Health and Education Ethiopia, Site Report No. 3. Metta, Eastern Hararge

**von Massow, F., A. Terefe, A. Bekele, S. Feyissa, T. Haile, A. Kidane Gebrehiwot, T. Koyra, A. Worku, and D. Zewdie** (1999) Oxfam Policy Department Micro Research: Health and Education Ethiopia, Site Report No. 4. Jijiga, Somali Region

**von Massow, F.** (1999) Oxfam Policy Department Micro Research: Health and Education Ethiopia Summary Report

## Ethiopian government policy documents:

Health Policy of the Transitional Government of Ethiopia (1993)

Education and Training Policy (1994)

National Population Policy of Ethiopia (1993)

National Policy on Ethiopian Women (1993)

Policy on HIV/AIDS of the Federal Democratic Republic of Ethiopia (1998)

**McGee, R., C. Robinson, and A. van Diesen** (1998) *Distant Targets: Making the 21ˢᵗ-Century Development Strategy Work,* Christian Aid

**Randel, J., T. German, and D. Ewing** (eds) (2000) *The Reality of Aid,* London: Earthscan

**Spandacini, B. and P. Nichols** (1998) 'Campaigning against female genital mutilation in Ethiopia using popular education', *Gender and Development* 6/2

**UNDP** *UNDP Human Development Reports* 1991, 1993, 1995, 1999

**UNFPA** (1999) *Six Billion: a Time for Choices,* New York: UNFPA

**van Diesen A., and K. Walker** (1999) *The Changing Face of Aid to Ethiopia,* Christian Aid publications

**von Massow, F.** '*"We are forgotten on earth"*: international development targets, poverty and gender in Ethiopia', *Gender and Development* 8/1

**World Bank** (1998/99) *World Development Report,* New York: Oxford University Press

# Appendix 1: Micro-research methodology

## Organisational structure

The health and education research and advocacy project was initiated and co-ordinated by the Health Adviser in the Oxfam GB Policy Department. The research was funded by Oxfam GB and implementation managed and co-ordinated by the Addis Ababa office of Oxfam GB in Ethiopia. The successful implementation of the research hinged on the support provided by Oxfam Ethiopia staff, PA and *kebele* representatives, and local government offices concerned with education, health, and agriculture.

The micro-research fieldwork took three months, from January to March 1999. The team included a team leader, two senior researchers and four assistant researchers, a senior statistician and one secretary, with a well-balanced combination of sex, age, and experience.

## Research tools and questionnaire content

The research, while aiming to maximise the input of experience, needs, and interests of various groups in the community, had specific objectives. This resulted in a methodology combining PRA[72] tools with a questionnaire format, which allowed for focused discussions on poverty, livelihoods, nutrition, health, reproductive health, and education. Working with single-sex focus groups of men, women, girls, and boys facilitated cross-referencing and comparisons between different gender and age perspectives, within the PRA data collected.

Time-line interviews were held with an elderly man and/or woman in each site. Their perceptions of trends in poverty, disease incidence, health-care provision, and schooling at various periods since Haile Selassie's regime provided an historical background for each site.

The qualitative information gathered during the PRA was substantiated and compared with data collected in a series of 35 household interviews, from which 30 were selected for analysis. Interviews were conducted with a questionnaire.

Finally government, private, and traditional providers of education and health services were interviewed, using prepared questionnaire formats. Responses from the community have been cross-referenced and compared with the views and statistics provided by providers of health and education services. This has created a useful picture of the barriers facing different groups in their attempts to gain access to health and education services.

Representatives of Peasant Associations, *kebeles*, and Elders worked on developing a Venn diagram identifying the most important local institutions and their problem-solving channels. Women were very under-represented in these sessions – except in Jijiga, when representatives of 'respected' women were asked to join the (all-male) Elders.

A market study of products and prices was conducted in the three rural sites, providing insights into the gender-determined and age-related division of labour in bulk and petty trading, and into prices and the cost of living.

## Site selection and fieldwork

Four sites were selected, including one urban slum, and three rural locations. The three rural sites were near to Oxfam regional offices in Delanta, North Wollo; Metta, Eastern Hararge; and Jijiga, Somali region. Two villages were visited in Jijiga, but the first attempt was abandoned, owing to bad weather and poor security conditions. The relative proximity of the sites to the Oxfam regional offices helped to prepare the communities for the research and to invite people to participate. An important criterion for site selection was that the communities had not participated in any PRA exercise previously. The team spent ten days in each site, except in Jijiga, where two days were spent in one site and six days in the second site.

Single-sex focus-group discussions took five days. Male researchers worked with the men and boys' groups, and female researchers worked with the women and girls. One of the main problems experienced by the researchers was how to probe further into the experience of individuals' poverty. The question of *what* to probe further also requires a constant overview of the purpose of the research. While the senior researchers for health and education undertook interviews with service providers, the assistant researchers did household interviews. It was agreed that men should not interview women, because a lot of personal information was required.

In Metta and Jijiga, the research was further complicated by the need to translate from Amharic into Orominya and Somali respectively. The key challenge for the researchers was to maintain control of the process and make sure that the information did not remain with the translators. One outcome of using translators for the research was in effect the provision of on-the-job training in PRA techniques and translation for about eight[73] women and men, some of whom will undoubtedly be employed by the Oxfam regional offices again.

## Participant selection

This was not a needs-assessment exercise. People were asked to participate to facilitate the communication of their views to decision-makers, within and outside Ethiopia, for the wider benefit of communities in Ethiopia living under similar circumstances.

Each community was informed about the number and age range of those needed for the PRA/focus-group discussions and was discouraged from recruiting couples, so that a larger number of households could be represented. In each site, two groups of 12 women, two groups of 12 men, and one group each of 12 girls and boys (aged 10–18) were involved. In the rural sites, villages were made up of between 70 to 170 households. So with approximately 48 women and men from different households participating, about 28-30 per cent of households of the village/s in the site participated in the research. In each site a meeting with the Elders and/or PA leaders was organised.

In Delanta the numbers of participants in the women's groups varied because of their many domestic and productive responsibilities. The research in Delanta also coincided with the first distribution of food aid in four months, and a major festival for which women had to prepare food. A total of about 300 people participated in the focus-group discussions in the five sites[74] visited.

The household survey was designed to include at least 30 household interviews, divided into three poverty categories: worst off, medium income, and better off. In each site 35 households were interviewed: 20 worst off, 10 medium income, and 5 better off. Since an important part of the household interview required intimate knowledge of women's reproductive health, about 70 per cent of respondents were women. A total of 140 or more (in some households husband and wife participated) participated in the household interviews.

Households with women of reproductive age and children of primary-school age were selected for interview. In Metta and Addis Ababa, 30 per cent of the households interviewed were headed by women; the comparable figures for Jijiga were 17 per cent and for Delanta 10 per cent. Most of them were in the worst-off category.

Providers of health and education services known to and used by women and men in the community were identified during the mapping exercise, which was the research team's very first contact with the community. Health and education professionals, parents' committees, Koran schoolteachers, trained and untrained traditional birth attendants, herbalists, traditional bonesetters and physiotherapists, priests and healers, drug stores and private practitioners were placed on the map and subsequently selected for interview. *Woreda* and zone health and education officials were also interviewed, and health and education statistics collected. Local government representatives and health personnel were predominantly male, as were teaching staff in the rural areas.

## Data processing and analysis

### PRA focus groups and service-provider questionnaires

The questionnaires were coded. Researchers took notes in Amharic and later transcribed their notes into English, with a margin for the codes and comments. A form, recording date, site, session, sex, and number of participants, was attached to the notes and filed according to session. The data were then entered in the computer.

### Household questionnaires

The senior statistician had in-depth discussion and feed-back sessions between sites with the team. Much of the data was of a descriptive nature, with many open-ended questions. The household questionnaire was translated by the team from English into Amharic, to reduce individual interpretations during interviews. Problems arose in data collection because most respondents had never been involved in a survey before and were not accustomed to the content and construction of the questions. They also survive in a very contradictory environment. Questions had to be explained, and the problems were compounded in Oromo and Somali regions, when the researchers had to work through translators. The time allocated for each site was not sufficient to allow for field editing and returning to households to verify responses. Despite these problems, the team was broadly satisfied with the outcome, and the data collected provide a good reference point and back-up, and a basis for comparative analysis for the data collected during the focus-group discussions and service-provider interviews.

## Methodology for the macro research

The research utilised a literature survey, a review of official statistics, and a review of policy and planning documents. Key individuals involved in planning, financing, and managing the health and education sector programmes at the levels of federal government, region, zone, and *woreda* were also interviewed. The research team visited the four regions involved in the micro research. Two donors, the World Bank and SIDA, long involved in the health and education sectors, were also interviewed.

# Appendix 2: Tabulated findings

**Table 3: Main health problems reported by communities in the four micro-research sites**

| Addis Ababa | Delanta | Metta | Jijiga |
|---|---|---|---|
| TB/HIV/AIDS[75] | Mogne Bagne[76] | 'Paralysis'[77] | TB |
| Hepatitis | Skin diseases | Scabies | |
| Diarrhoea | Diarrhoea | Diarrhoea | Diarrhoea |
| Typhoid | Typhoid | Gastritis | |
| Abortion | Pregnancy-associated | Gynaecological | Anaemia in pregnancy |
| | Excessive bleeding on delivery | Excessive bleeding on delivery | Excessive bleeding on delivery |
| | | FGM (infibulation) | FGM (infibulation) |
| | | Early pregnancy | |
| Common cold | Common cold | Tonsilitis/RTI | Coughs and colds |
| | Eye diseases | Injury due to accidents and violence[78] | Tonsillitis and uvelectomy[79] |
| | Ear aches (insect) | Swollen body - children | |

(Source: Site reports 1 – 4 and Oxfam Micro Research Health and Education Summary Report, 1999)

**Table 4: Percentage of pregnant women testing positive for HIV**

| Place | 1992/93 | 1997 |
|---|---|---|
| **Urban (ante-natal care)** | | |
| **Addis Ababa** | 11.2 | |
| Kazanchis Health Centre | 16.7 | |
| Tekle Haimanot Health Centre | | 18.5 |
| Gulele Health Centre | | 20.0 |
| Kefitegna 23 Health Centre | | 14.1 |
| Akaki factory workers | | 12.7 |
| **Metu** | 10.7 | |
| **Dire Dawa** | 12.3 | |
| **Baher Dar** | 13.0 | |
| **Gambella Hospital** | | 12.7 |

| Place | 1992/93 | 1997 |
|---|---|---|
| **Rural (general population)** | | |
| Seya Debir (North Shoa) | 1.3 | |
| Shola Gebeya (North Shoa) | 6.6 | |
| Enda Mariam Kanaro (Tigray) | 0.0 | |
| Ayuba (Arsi) | 0.2 | |
| Raytu (Bale) | 1.0 | |
| Beneste (South Omo) | 2.0 | |
| **Country-wide (MOH estimates)** | **3.2** | **7.4** |

(Source: MOH 1998 pp. 4 and 5)

**Table 5: Health Sector Development Programme planned budgets (by component, in Birrs)**

| Component | Planned Capital | Recurrent | Total planned | Percent | Capital to recurrent ratio |
|---|---|---|---|---|---|
| Service delivery and quality of care | 267,105,000 | 2,044,756,600 | 2,311,861,600 | 51.4 | 0.13 |
| Health facility rehabilitation/ expansion | 1,040,457,000 | 196,164,400 | 1,236,621,400 | 27.5 | 5.30 |
| Human resources development | 65,735,800 | 71,971,100 | 137,706,900 | 3.1 | 0.91 |
| Pharmaceutical services | 185,008,100 | 453,719,600 | 638,727,700 | 14.2 | 0.41 |
| Information/ Education/ Communication | 20,644,500 | 36,317,710 | 56,962,210 | 1.3 | 0.57 |
| Health sector management MIS | 23,090,700 | 62,635,500 | 85,726,200 | 1.9 | 0.37 |
| Monitoring and evaluation | 16,345,000 | 8,838,000 | 25,183,000 | 0.6 | 1.85 |
| Health care financing | 1,547,200 | 5,934,400 | 7,481,600 | 0.2 | 0.26 |
| Total | 1,619,933,300 | 2,880,337,310 | 4,500,270,610 | 100% | 0.56 |

(Source: Health Sector Development Programme 1998)

The financing modalities anticipated to cover the costs of the HSDP are shown in Table 6. The government committed itself to financing 55 per cent of total health expenditure. It is expected that external aid will cover 43 per cent, and user fees 2 per cent.

**Table 6: Indicative financing plan (in millions of Birrs)**

| Programme costs financed by | 1998/99 | 1999/00 | 2000/01 | Total | % of total expenditure |
|---|---|---|---|---|---|
| Government | 447 | 487 | 1,840 | 2,774 | 55% |
| User fees | 20 | 20 | 64 | 103 | 2% |
| External aid | 310 | 527 | 1,289 | 2,125 | 43% |
| Total | 777 | 1,034 | 3,192 | 5,002 | |

(Source: Health Sector Development Programme 1998)

**Table 7: HSDP allocation for different regions by category of expenditure (in Birrs)**

| Region | Authorised HSDP allocation | Capital | Recurrent | Total planned | Contingency |
|---|---|---|---|---|---|
| Tigrai | 346,864,000 | 70,702,681 | 241,474,919 | 312,177,600 | 34,686,400 |
| Afar | 228,200,000 | 104,440,077 | 100,704,100 | 205,144,177 | 23,055,823 |
| Amhara | 876,288,000 | 375,537,700 | 413,121,400 | 788,659,100 | 87,628,900 |
| Oromia | 1,154,692,000 | 353,064,000 | 686,581,960 | 1,039,645,960 | 115,046,040 |
| Somali | 342,300,000 | 140,350,360 | 167,729,700 | 308,080,060 | 34,219,940 |
| Benshangul Gumuz | 173,432,000 | 58,015,800 | 96,865,500 | 154,881,300 | 18,550,700 |
| SNNPR | 725,676,000 | 253,721,500 | 399,117,400 | 652,838,900 | 72,837,100 |
| Gambella | 127,792,000 | 53,058,000 | 61,954,800 | 115,012,800 | 12,779,200 |
| Harari | 82,152,000 | 21,221,400 | 51,796,700 | 73,018,100 | 9,133,900 |
| Addis Ababa | 333,172,000 | 68,995,000 | 231,839,600 | 300,834,600 | 32,337,400 |
| Dire Dawa | 173,432,000 | 46,495,400 | 109,281,300 | 155,776,700 | 17,655,300 |
| Centre/MOH | 438,000,000 | 74,330,600 | 319,869,400 | 394,200,000 | 43,800,000 |
| *Total* | *5,002,000,000* | *1,619,932,518* | *2,880,336,779* | *4,500,269,297* | *501,730,703* |

(Source: Health Sector Development Programme 1998)

Tigrai's 77 per cent planned expenditure on recurrent costs is similar to that of Addis Ababa, Harari, Dire Dawa, and the federal MOH-run services. Regions such as Afar, Amhara, Somali, and Gambella spend 49 per cent, 52 per cent, and 54 per cent respectively on recurrent costs, significantly less than the other regions.

**Table 8: Share of recurrent expenditures of total planned budget**

| Region | Recurrent as % of total expenditure |
|---|---|
| Tigrai | 77% |
| Afar | 49 |
| Amhara | 52 |
| Oromia | 66 |
| Somali | 54 |
| Benshangul Gumuz | 63 |
| SNNPR | 61 |
| Gambella | 54 |
| Harari | 71 |
| Addis Ababa | 77 |
| Dire Dawa | 70 |
| Centre/MOH | 81 |
| Total | 0.64 |

Note: the above calculation excludes contingency plans.

**Table 9: Ratios of health worker to population in regions of Ethiopia**

|  | Physician/ Population | Pharmacist/ population | Nurse/ population | Health Assistant/ population | Population per hospital bed |
|---|---|---|---|---|---|
| **Tigrai** | 39,068 | 559,980 | 6,899 | 2,687 | 3,240 |
| **Afar** | 75,676 | 1,135,149 | 25,798 | 8,665 | 17,464 |
| **Amhara**[81] | 59,889 | 616,361 | 22,144 | 6,431 | 14,376 |
| **Oromia** | 55,052 | 607,248 | 19,860 | 6,254 | 12,595 |
| **Somali** | 79,996 | 1,146,620 | 24,396 | 10,298 | 9,828 |
| **Benshangul** | 17,002 | 123,270 | 6,241 | 2,211 | 1,941 |
| **SNNP** | 43,479 | 554,367 | 21,487 | 6,564 | 10,681 |
| **Gambella** | 12,177 | 38,967 | 3,542 | 1,464 | 2,051 |
| **Harari** | 3,392 | 47,491 | 2,064 | 1,024 | 414 |
| **Addis** | 11,176 | 82,624 | 4,123 | 3,672 | 2,509 |
| **Dire Dawa** | 8,320 | 91,520 | 3,813 | 2,640 | 1,551 |

(Source: Health Sector Development Programme 1998)

Tigrai, Amhara, Oromia, and SNNP are the regions with highest population densities. The regions with lowest population densities, Afar and Somali, have the highest population/health worker ratios and an extremely low drug-store availability, compared with other regions. These figures show the poverty of the health infrastructure in these regions.

**Table 10: Population per health centre and health station in regions of Ethiopia**

| Region | Population per Health Centre | Population per Health Station |
|---|---|---|
| **Tigray** | 176,836 | 17,591 |
| **Afar** | 227,030 | 19,572 |
| **Amhara** | 264,155 | 21,346 |
| **Oromia** | 263,674 | 15,427 |
| **Somali** | 343,986 | 38,650 |
| **Benshangul** | 123,271 | 6,755 |
| **SNNP** | 133,583 | 24,860 |
| **Gambella** | 48,709 | 4,236 |
| **Harari** | 142,474 | 5,480 |
| **Addis** | 128,527 | 6,824 |
| **Dire Dawa** | 137,281 | 10,560 |

(Source: Ministry of Health, 1998)

## Table 11: Infant mortality and life expectancy by region

| Region | Infant mortality | Under-5 Mortality | % of children underweight | Life expectancy at birth[81] |
|---|---|---|---|---|
| **Urban** | | | | |
| **Addis Ababa** | 78 | 109 | 45.4% | 58.4 |
| **Harare** | 113 | 166 | 27.8% | 51.4 |
| **Dire Dawa** | 115 | 168 | 42.5% | 51.1 |
| **Rural** | | | | |
| **Tigrai** | 123 | 161 | 57% | 49.6 |
| **Amhara** | 115 | 170 | 55.6% | 50.8 |
| **Oromia** | 118 | 173 | 37.4% | 50.4 |
| **Benshangul Gumuz** | 140 | 206 | 43.8% | 46.8 |
| **Gambella** | 96 | 142 | 33.4% | 54.2 |
| **SNNP** | 128 | 189 | 49.6% | 48.6 |
| **Afar** | 118 | 174 | 39% | 50.3 |
| **Somali** | 96 | 137 | 41.2% | 54.8 |

(Source: CSA statistical bulletin 1999)

## Table 12: Rural-urban distribution of schools by level and region (1998/99)

| Region | Total Primary | Total Secondary | No. schools Primary (rural) | % of total | No. schools secondary (rural) | % of total |
|---|---|---|---|---|---|---|
| **Tigray** | 811 | 26 | 683 | 84.2 | 0 | 0 |
| **Afar** | 101 | 4 | 74 | 73.3 | 0 | 0 |
| *Amhara*[82] | 2,819 | 84 | 2,548 | 90.4 | 9 | 10.7 |
| *Oromia* | 4,200 | 128 | 3,604 | 85.8 | 2 | 1.6 |
| *Somali* | 167 | 3 | 129 | 77.2 | 0 | 0 |
| **Benishangul–Gumuz** | 257 | 9 | 237 | 92.2 | 0 | 0 |
| **SNNP** | 2,228 | 81 | 1,968 | 88.3 | 10 | 12.3 |
| **Gambella** | 123 | 6 | 113 | 91.9 | 3 | 50 |
| **Harari** | 44 | 3 | 22 | 50.0 | 0 | 0 |
| *Addis Ababa* | 248 | 41 | 1 | 0.04 | 0 | 0 |
| **Dire Dawa** | 53 | 4 | 25 | 47.2 | 0 | 0 |
| *Ethiopia* | *1,1051* | *386* | *9,404* | *85.1* | *24* | *6.2* |

(Source: Education Statistics Annual Abstract, 1998/99)

Of the research sites, Somali region is the worst-serviced in terms of rural secondary schools (none), and new primary-school construction since 1994/5 (none). Between 1994/5 and 1998/9 there was a 10 per cent increase in new schools constructed in Amhara region, a 15 per cent increase in Oromia, and an 11 per cent increase in Addis Ababa. This is, however, no indicator of difference in the quality of service provision.

**Table 13: Rural–urban dimensions of primary enrolment, 1997/98, by region**

| Region | Urban Boys | Urban Girls | Total | Rural Boys | Rural Girls | Total |
|---|---|---|---|---|---|---|
| Tigray | 83,204 | 73,212 | 156,416 | 139,089 | 102,438 | 241,527 |
| Afar | 4,564 | 3,624 | 8,188 | 4,476 | 2,127 | 6,603 |
| Amhara | 152,651 | 151,275 | 303,926 | 440,117 | 316,043 | 756,160 |
| Oromia | 348,855 | 250,338 | 599,193 | 820,832 | 290,893 | 1,111,725 |
| Somali | 16,984 | 6,858 | 23,842 | 27,753 | 10,242 | 37,995 |
| Ben.- Gumuz | 9,682 | 5,712 | 15,394 | 40,960 | 16,371 | 57,331 |
| SNNPR | 170,477 | 109,876 | 280,353 | 743,248 | 307,592 | 1,050,840 |
| Gambella | 3,728 | 2,784 | 6,512 | 17,471 | 8,589 | 26,060 |
| Harari | 7,988 | 7,323 | 15,311 | 4,145 | 1,372 | 5,517 |
| Addis Ababa | 171,005 | 186,579 | 357,584 | 88 | 57 | 145 |
| Dire Dawa | 13,882 | 12,669 | 26,551 | 2,866 | 631 | 3,497 |
| Total | 983,020 | 810,250 | 1,793,270 | 2,241,045 | 1,056,355 | 3,297,400 |

(Source: Education Statistics Annual Abstract, 1997/98)

**Table 14: Total budget allocated to education and capital budget 1994/95 to 1996/97**

| Level | 1994/95 Birr millions Total budget | Capital budget | 1995/96 Birr millions Total budget | Capital budget | 1996/97 Birr millions Total budget | Capital budget |
|---|---|---|---|---|---|---|
| **Primary** | 811.4 | 209.4 | 846.4 | 206.4 | 804.2 | 158.34 |
| **Secondary** | 131.1 | 26.6 | 136.89 | 28.0 | 186.3 | 78.7 |
| **Tertiary and others** | 163.2 | 72.7 | 355.93 | 106.6 | 506.1 | 116.47 |
| **Total education budget** | 1,297.2 | 411.9 | 1,339.22 | 393.9 (441.86)[a] | 1,496.6 | 480.39 (429.47)[b] |
| **Total government budget** | 9,964.6 | 4,595.2 | 9,667.35 | 3,966.41 | 10,923 | 4,835.1 |
| **Share of education in total (%)** | 13.0% | 9.0 | 13.9% | 9.9 | 13.7% | 9.9 |

(Source: MOE, Planning and Programming Panel)

# Appendix 3
# Case study 1: Cherkos, Kebele 24, Addis Ababa

## Poverty, livelihoods, and nutrition

The ranking exercise in Cherkos told us that about 70% of the community are classified as the 'worst-off'. For the vast majority of families, this means that they do not have sufficient income to cover their basic food requirements, basic health-care costs, or the costs of sending all their children to primary school. Table 15 shows how women and men in Cherkos define poverty and relative well-being.

## Factors contributing to poverty

Cherkos is an area strongly associated with its market and with the military camp that it surrounds. The economic status of the area is closely linked to the fate of the Ethiopian army. At the downfall of Mengistu's Derg regime in 1991, a significant proportion of his army was demobilised, resulting in high male unemployment, and a reduction at the same time in custom for women's food and drink trade and the sex trade. In addition there are many older military pensioners in the area, and high male and youth unemployment. Many families depend on women's daily petty trading for a living.

## Table 15: How the poor classify poverty in Kebele 24

| 'worst-off' households | 'medium' households | 'better-off' households |
|---|---|---|
| *71 % of the sample* | *21% of the sample* | *8% of the sample* |
| • Large family size (10+). | • Married couple, no children, with low insecure income (musician), | • Small family size. |
| • Small pension (less than 50 birr per month). | • They have (his) small pension, which they supplement with other jobs. | • He has an adequate pension, enough for the family. |
| • A very sick head of household (male). | • They have support from other sources (children). | • He/she has a well-paid job. |
| • The husband has died or left the household. | • Pensioned but with a large family. | • Someone who is permanently employed. |
| • W/ro Teitu: *'I am a mother of 7, my husband died. The oldest is in government school, the others are at home. My children have food one day and not the next.'* | • The husband or wife has permanent employment but only a small income (e.g. the husband is a zabanya). | • Both the husband and wife work. |
| • Lack adequate food and clothing and treatment when sick. | • Good health, ability to work and be active. | • He has his own house. |
| • No reliable job (both husband and wife). | • Some men have trades (carpenter, weaver, tailor) but have no permanent work in the market and do not get regular work. | • He/she has good pay. |
| • Loss of means of income due to age and/or sickness. Families surviving on a daily income e.g. women's petty trade – fuel wood, preparing and selling berberri, washing clothes, brewing the local beer, 'tella'. | | • He/she has support from children (some overseas). |
| • Widows looking after orphaned children. | | |
| • The family size is smaller. | | |

(Source: Focus-group discussions)

60

The population of Kebele 24 is around 15,000, and has grown. With the increasing job losses and a drop in incomes, and no serious investment in poverty reduction, health care, water and sanitation, or primary education services, the prospects for the next generation are bleak. One woman predicted that there would be no one left. They are dying, they said, but it's a slow and miserable way to live and die. The key causes and effects of poverty highlighted by the participants (women and men) were as follows.

• Unemployment
• Poor health
• Shortage of water
• Poor environmental sanitation: rubbish, no toilets, overflowing public latrines, open drains
• Bad infrastructure: no access roads, poor sanitation, irregular water supply, contaminated water
• Overcrowded housing
• Large family size (86 per cent of the 'worst-off households' in the survey had 4–8 children)
• Security problems: street violence (boys), fear of abuse and rape (girls and women)
• Delinquency, drug abuse, and alcoholism (mostly boys, young men)
• Lack of employment perspectives for young men and women
• *'Mental unrest and disturbance amongst young people, as a result of unemployment'* (a main health problem raised by young girls).

An older man in the group explained: *'Many of the population in this Kebele are very, very poor. In old days most of the people had large income. Now they do not even have enough to get food. When we say better off here, we mean people who get enough food. Categorising very poor indicate here for those who do not get food once a day.'*

## Livelihood patterns

In Cherkos, there is a significant number of army pensioners whose families wholly or in part depend on their pension for an income. However, there are also many families with a very small pension or no pension, and a significant proportion of households, maybe more than 30%, are headed by women. Some people are forced to beg for a living. Livelihoods are vulnerable, varying with fluctuations in the agricultural calendar, the rainy and dry seasons, festivals and holidays. As a rule, however, women's earning power is less than men's. A high proportion of households is dependent on women's low incomes, a contributory factor to the level of poverty in the area. Table 16 shows broad categories of livelihoods by gender and the factors affecting income levels over the year.

In the dry season (December to May) there is a higher demand for daily labour and construction workers. The harvest seasons (December to February) are important for women traders, as prices are lower and there is wider range of products available to sell. During this time some men trade in larger quantities of grains and chickpeas, selling to smaller traders.

Income levels decrease dramatically during the rainy months from June to September. Everyone is less mobile, because of heavy rains and flooding. The agricultural prices are higher, and there is little or no construction. Business and trading are depressed. In June students compete with adults for work. In July and August there is no work in the coffee-cleaning plant, an important source of income for women and girls. All these factors affect the livelihoods of women and men and children and reduce the availability and circulation of money in the community. This coincides with the season of high expenditure needs, and therefore borrowing. School fees, exercise books, and uniforms have to be purchased in September, which is also the month of Ethiopian New Year celebrations. The rains bring an increase in the incidence of illness, and the need to seek and pay for cures is at its highest.

## Incomes and food security

Many households right in the centre of Addis are seriously lacking in food most of the year: 85% of worst-off and 43% of medium households report difficulty in maintaining adequate nutrition. *'Absolutely unbearable and difficult condition has come about in the last four years. Virtually the people have little or nothing to eat'* (men's group). Two things became clear from our household survey: incomes in the worst-off and medium households are too low to buy adequate food supplies for large families; and almost all income in worst-off and medium families is spent on food.

The women's group said that most people eat 'shurro' (a sauce made with finely ground chickpeas) and njera, and that they lack fruit and vegetables in their diet and rarely eat meat. Some make the shurro with 'guaya', a plant known for its poisonous properties. People who eat too much of it become lame and permanently disabled. They eat it because it is very cheap. In the household survey, 95% of worst-off and 100% of medium households gave 'insufficient income' as the cause of inadequate nutrition for children.

**Table 16: Factors affecting seasonal fluctuations in income by source of income and gender**

| Source of income | Gender | Factors affecting the market | | Season | |
| | | Increase in income | Decrease in income | | |
| --- | --- | --- | --- | --- | --- |
| Petty trade in agricultural products | Mostly Women | | Fasting | Hidar | (Nov) |
| Charcoal production & sale | Women & men | Christmas Weddings & Epiphany Easter New Year | | Tahisas Tir<br><br>Miyazia Meskerem | (Dec) (Jan.)<br><br>(April) (Sept) |
| Petty trading Beer/alcohol producers Baking njera Producing berberri | Women & girls | Harvests<br><br>Chilli harvest | | Tahisas Tir<br><br>Tikmt | (Dec) (Jan)<br><br>(Oct) |
| Bulk purchases for resale | Mostly men, some women | Harvests | | Tahisas/Tir | (Dec/Jan) |
| Petty trading Food/alcohol production | Mostly women | | No purchasers after Easter | Ginbot | (May) |
| Coffee -cleaning plant Daily labour | Mostly women | | No beans | Hamiley/Nehassey | (July/Aug.) |
| Daily labour Construction work Transporting goods | Mostly men | | Heavy rains & flooding | Seney – Meskerem | (June – Sept.) |
| Petty trading | Women and girls | | Heavy rains & flooding | Seney – Meskerem | (June – Sept.) |

(Source: focus-group discussions)

A staggering 90% of worst-off households, and 50% of medium households, reported failing to maintain adequate nutrition for their children. In the worst-off households, 25% of children were reported to be showing the signs of malnutrition. This may well be an underestimate, as mothers are reluctant to admit to what they see as a failure on their part. In one household interviewed, it was the 16-year-old daughter who 'reminded' her mother that the clinic had said that her little brother's illness was related to lack of food. Her mother had been saying that none of her children suffered from nutrition-related problems.

The most difficult period is the rainy season, when incomes are low and food stocks run out. Families adjust their diet and the number of meals they eat per day. In worst-off households 10% reported only drinking water, 40% reported just eating maize or potatoes, and 20% just eat 'kita', a local bread; 50% of the medium-poverty group and 20% of the worst-off reported eating roasted cereals ('kollo' or 'nifro', a type of bread). Parents eat less, so that their children can eat what little there is. Some adults manage on just coffee in the morning and water at night for several days. Some women said: *'If he is a considerate husband he would eat with his wife, but there are those who eat all the food by themselves.'* Women believe that they can manage longer without food than men. They also said that girls *'can endure hunger better than boys'*. Some girls give their breakfast to their brothers before going to school. *'In hungry seasons children even steal food and money to buy food,'* said one mother.

Finally, during the focus-group discussions and service-provider interviews, there were allusions made to men's drinking and socialising, and to young boys indulging in alcohol, cigarettes, and drugs. The survey has not extended to investigating the details of men's and boys income and expenditure habits, nor who controls men's access to income for socialising, including extra-marital sexual activity (source: Kebele leaders). This may well be a circulation of money outside the household budget and merits further enquiry.

## Health

### Water and sanitation

**Water:** According to the PRA there are about 15 owners of private taps in the community, and people buy water at around 0.15 cents per 'baldi'. Most households interviewed said that it takes an average of 20 to 30 minutes to collect water. Several participants were concerned about the quality of the water, believing it is contaminated because the piping system is so old and rotten.

There are no significant seasonal differences in access to water; however, water often has to be collected in the evening, as the supply can be cut off in the day. It is mostly women and girls who collect and carry water, although boys from the poorer households also undertake this task from time to time. This is significant not only because of the extra burden placed on women's and girls' time and strength, but because it is simply unsafe to go out in the evening. There was a lot of talk of abuse and rape of young women, and the Kebele officials said that people were most vulnerable to muggings, stone-throwing, theft, and beatings between 7.00 p.m. and 9.00 p.m.

**Sanitation:** The sanitation situation in the Kebele is appalling, with open, overflowing sewers, and streams of human and other waste running down the streets and pathways between the tightly packed dwellings. The whole area is littered with rubbish. Few households have toilets. Some bore a hole from their houses into the underground concrete waste pipes and pour their waste down them, blocking them up further. Other households have a bucket or other container as a toilet and pour its contents into the open gutters in the streets.

In the Derg's time some public toilets were constructed as part of Kebele-organised community development. These ran into disrepair, and were full or overflowing and filthy at the time of the study. One neighbourhood has formed an association of 50 households with the assistance of the Oxfam-funded NGO VCH. Members contributed to the costs of having a tanker come and empty the latrines standing in their midst. They pay 5.00 Birr per month to use the latrines. Two women are employed to hold the keys and to clean the latrines.

The Kebele has built two more blocks of latrines, using contributions from the community. These are not yet in use. No other actions to address this very acute problem are being taken by government or NGOs. Hopes had been raised by the prospect of possible funding for a roads-improvement and urban sanitation programme, but the community is too poor to raise the required contributions in cash to the World Bank Ethiopian Social Rehabilitation and Development Fund.

### Main diseases identified by men and women

The Kebele is very congested. The insanitary conditions described above are insupportable and are causing serious environmental health problems. Waste matter and other dirt are dumped along the road or in any open space. Unbalanced diets, poor housing, and the cold exacerbate the problems. Diarrhoea was reported as a serious health problem, mainly affecting children under the age of five, who also get typhoid. A TTBA interviewed said that the causes of disease in this area are filth, lack of toilets, and inability of the community and the government to address these issues.

The incidence of diseases peaks during the rains, when sanitation deteriorates further, there is a shortage of work, a problem compounded by low incomes, and little or no food. The incidence of diarrhoea, colds, and respiratory problems including TB increases considerably. *These problems are particularly serious among women petty traders in the market. You can see them coughing whenever the weather changes,'* said one man. Women suffer from umbilical hernias, mainly caused by overwork and carrying and/or lifting heavy loads. They are treated by TBAs.

Most of the health problems identified during the focus-group discussions and from the household survey were similar to those identified by the drug-store owner and the private clinic, and to the top ten diseases reported by the health centre for 1998 (see Table 18).

63

**Table 17: Major diseases and health problems identified by men's and women's focus-group discussions**

| Women's group | Men's group | Youth groups |
|---|---|---|
| TB (AIDS)* | TB* | TB* |
| Hepatitis* | Abdominal complications | HIV/AIDS* |
| Diarrhoea* (under 5) | Diarrhoea* (jardia common) | Common cold* |
| Typhoid* | Abortion* (young women and girls) | Diarrhoea* |
| Asthma | Common cold* | Mental unrest and disturbance |
| Liver problems | Diabetes | Unwanted pregnancy and abortions |
| | Typhoid – contaminated water | |
| | Asthma – air pollution | |
| | HIV/AIDS Venereal disease | |

(Note: those marked * are the four most prevalent problems identified.)

**Table 18: Top ten diseases reported by Kebele 09 Health Centre, Woreda 21 (1997/1998)**

| | Diagnosis | Number | Percentage |
|---|---|---|---|
| 1 | Acute upper-respiratory infections | 2500 | 12.76 |
| 2 | Bronchopneumonia | 2068 | 10.55 |
| 3 | Infections of the skin and subcutaneous tissue | 1630 | 8.32 |
| 4 | Gastritis and Duodenitis | 1350 | 6.89 |
| 5 | Other Helminths | 1317 | 6.72 |
| 6 | Hypertrophy of Tonsillitis | 907 | 4.63 |
| 7 | Other diseases of reproductive system | 825 | 4.21 |
| 8 | Infections of kidney | 635 | 3.24 |
| 9 | Gastroenteritis and colitis (4 weeks – 2 years) | 594 | 3.02 |
| 10 | Muscular rheumatism and arthritis | 585 | 2.98 |
| *Total* | | *12411* | *63.32* |

(Source: Cherkos health centre Kebele 09, Woreda 21. Note that these records reflect the incidence of illness of those, from the whole woreda, and neighbouring woredas, who seek treatment at the health centre. Many in Kebele 24 do not have access for a variety of reasons: see 'Health services' below.)

### Reproductive-health problems

The girls' group linked mental unrest among young unemployed males to their deviant behaviour, resulting in unwanted pregnancies and STDs among young girls. Girls are reportedly subjected to violence and rape, and many resort to abortion. The resultant fear and lack of security, they said, had affected their education and their health. Young boys are more affected by other forms of street violence: *'There are lots of young people (male) who have been wounded and killed due to urban violence,'* said the women.

The men's group included abortion as one of the four main health problems. A private clinic said: *'Abortion is one of the most important health hazards affecting our sisters. They are dying, and those who escape death end up having permanent damage.'*

According to both men and women, the victims of TB and HIV/AIDS are young men between the ages of 15 and 40. People believe that boys more than girls are affected; they said that they die sooner because they smoke and drink a lot. TB of the 'samba' (lung TB) is considered a nickname for HIV/AIDS in this Kebele. They know that it is AIDS, because the TB treatment should work but doesn't. They said, *'They get very thin, they cough and there is diarrhoea, many people die.'*

Young girls said they need reproductive-health education. The boys' youth group identified sex education as one of their basic health-education needs.

**Circumcision:** Although some TBAs stopped performing female circumcision three years ago in response to health education, circumcision of boys and of girls is still performed. The most common form of female circumcision in Kebele 24 is the removal of the tip of the clitoris. There were strongly differing views on the practice in the women's group, between those who believed it should stop and those who were insistent on circumcising their daughters.

**Antenatal care:** The majority of women in the household survey reported that they use antenatal services: 75% from the worst-off group, 86% from the medium group, and 100% from the better-off group. During their last pregnancy, 56% of worst-off, 29% of medium, and 67% of better-off reported having health problems. The main problems were related to malnutrition, including anaemia and miscarriage. The worst-off families have a very poor diet, and women tend to give what food there is to the children. Antenatal care is free, so the majority of the women in the worst-off group (72%) go to the government clinic and hospital for treatment when they are sick during pregnancy.

**Delivery:** Women in Kebele 24 do not have a maternity centre nearby. They deliver at home, at Kebele 18 health centre, or at government hospitals. Whereas 52% of women from the worst-off, and 43% from the medium-poverty categories delivered at home, all in the better-off category gave birth in a hospital or government health centre. Of the home deliveries, 48% in worst-off households were attended by an untrained TBA, a neighbour, or a relative. All women in better-off households were assisted by a doctor or a nurse during birth. In the worst-off group, 38% reported having problems after delivery; 40% of those reported heavy bleeding, and 20% anaemia.

It must be noted that a significant proportion of women in the worst-off and medium groups still give birth at home, and that these groups report problems during pregnancy and after birth. These are high-risk deliveries, taking place in overcrowded and insanitary conditions, attended by ill-equipped and untrained people.

**Family planning:** The health centre provides family-planning services free of charge.

Mothers going for antenatal care and other MCH services are the target group for family-planning education. Note that men and youth are thus not reached by family planning or reproductive-health education.

According to the survey, a very small percentage of women is using family planning. There appears to be a relationship between use of family planning and income. While 74% of worst-off and 80% of the medium households do not use family planning, 67% of better-off families do. About 30% of the worst-off households are headed by women; however, they may still have partners.

Family planning also needs to be differentiated by users. W/ro. Mitikie, a TBA, said that the number of women whom she was called to assist during delivery had declined. She thought that one of the reasons was that prostitutes are increasingly using condoms to protect themselves from HIV/AIDS infection, thus at the same time protecting themselves from unwanted pregnancy.

A widow, and mother of eight, said that she would have limited the number of children if she had known what it was leading her to. Having eight children, she is unable to satisfy their needs. They are not fed adequately, they do not have the necessary materials for school, and they do not get access to proper health care.

## Health services

**Types of service:** The types of service available include health centre; hospital; private clinics; illegal private practitioners; drug stores; traditional healers; Ato Mamo, famous traditional healer; Traditional Birth Attendants (trained and untrained); Wogeishas (traditional physiotherapists/bonesetters); holy waters (church); home treatment. The nearest government health centre in Kebele 09 provides the following services.

- Health education
- Antenatal care
- Postnatal care
- Family planning
- Vaccination and immunisation
- Consultation
- Laboratory
- Emergencies
- Pharmacy
- Leprosy and TB programme
- STD programme.

However, due to the complexities of the exemption system, and to the fact that, for those who do have an exemption paper, there are no medicines for treatment, many from Kebele 24 are discouraged from using the facility. The health centre is seriously oversubscribed, with a doctor:population ratio of 1:197,895. Participants complained about the long queues and the preferential treatment given to paying users or those known personally to staff/guards. Many use home treatment or traditional healers, or just go without treatment. Women say that all services except the bonesetter, the TBA, and the health centre provide medicine.

Women are aware of reproductive-health education services at the health centre, but men are not. It is possible, therefore, that, unless men come for STD treatment, they will not access any reproductive-health education. Given the level of sexual promiscuity, early pregnancies, rape, and HIV/AIDS in the area, described by all participants, it would seem essential that men and boys should be reached by health education. The men's group was aware of the STD clinic at the health centre, but women were not. This may also be an indicator that women do not recognise and treat STDs, and men do. Many men just go to the drug store and treat themselves. Women say that in the case of an emergency they go to all health facilities except the church. Men did not mention emergencies.

**Health-seeking behaviour and accessibility of treatment:** Women and men will choose to go to a government health centre if the complaint is serious, but they need a referral to a government hospital (e.g. for TB). Men believe that women prefer traditional healers, while they themselves chose to go to the health centre. Women were more particular about matching the complaint to the service provider. They said that it is good to go to hospital when children have diarrhoea and for car accidents. But they are more confident in traditional healers' ability to treat hepatitis, almaze (a sometimes fatal skin-rash, caused by the bite of an insect called almaze), STDs, and tonsillitis.

Most households in the worst-off group reported low cost as the main reason for selecting the location of treatment. These households have no money to make a choice. The youth groups, especially the girls, reported having home treatment because their mothers could not afford anything else. They seek treatment elsewhere only when the condition is much worse. Women do not go to the clinic unless they are seriously ill. Distance is the second most important factor for this group. Most cannot afford transport. The sick need to go by taxi, which costs about Birr 21.00 (US$ 2.69).

There were a significant number of complaints from the worst-off and better-off groups alike about staff attitudes and discrimination at government health facilities.

**Affordability:** All focus groups reported that they could not afford to go to government health services. This was confirmed by health-service providers, including private clinics and drug stores, who said that they sometimes treated the very poor for nothing or at reduced cost. The situation was becoming impossible. Even TB treatment was too expensive, despite the fact that it is free, because of transport costs and the cost of nutritious food. In the household survey, 84% of worst-off households reported that health care was unaffordable, and the remaining 16% said it was 'affordable with a struggle' — i.e. they had to reduce food consumption, or had less cash available for school costs. A serious illness in the household was one of the reasons given for dropping out of school.

In theory, a paper giving exemption from user fees, obtained from the Kebele, should provide the patient with free diagnosis and treatment. In practice, the health centre has inadequate medical supplies and there is no medication for treatment. In addition, the Kebele is charging 5.00 Birr per exemption paper (which normally carries no charge), to cover community contributions to a World Bank part-funded project (The Ethiopian Social Rehabilitation and Development Fund) for the building of a maternity unit in a neighbouring Kebele. In effect, this means that the very poorest are being asked to contribute to investments in health-care infrastructure which they are least likely to use, or to forfeit access to an exemption form.

People also said that there was a very bureaucratic and time-consuming process to get the paper. The poor have a long working day, especially poor women, and do not have spare time. Participants therefore said that it was not worth applying for an exemption paper. For traditional health services, people have to pay up to Birr 20.00 (US$2.56) for a visit to the wogeisha or to have an untrained TBA attend their delivery. Sometimes these services are provided to very poor households free of charge or at reduced rates.

Some people reported borrowing money to cover health costs (at interest rates of up to 50%), selling assets like jewellery, furniture, or radios, and necessary possessions such as winter coats and beds. In some cases neighbours made a collection to help someone to get health care.

**Quality of health care:** The youth groups preferred private clinics to government services, because they felt they were diagnosed properly and listened to. People felt that government health–service staff have a negative attitude to the poor and do not treat them as well as they treat the better-off.

Young participants said that they were at the mercy of health-centre staff who use re-useable needles. The youth group were very conscious of the dangers of government and traditional health practitioners using used needles and razor blades.

There were several criticisms about staff attitudes in government health facilities, including their treating poor people '*like dogs*' (male participant). The girls' group and the women also gave the health centre a very low rating for staff attitude to the poor. The health centre is underfunded and has a shortage of staff, especially of appropriately qualified staff. They are aware that they are unable to provide the sort of service they would wish for.

Women were concerned about cost, the distance to the health centre, and having access to a 24-hour service. The availability of medicine was extremely important to all groups. Both adult groups gave availability of medicine at government health facilities a low score. This was also raised as a main problem by health-service providers, in terms of both availability and affordability for the poor.

Finally, waiting time was a crucial aspect of quality health-service delivery. All groups gave the health centre and government hospitals the lowest score for waiting time. Given that patients from the poorest households, especially women, are brought to a government facility when the condition has deteriorated considerably, a long wait can make the difference between life and death.

Good diagnosis and trained medical staff were important to most groups. For this reason, one girl said, it was good to go to a private clinic: '*because they ask you what is wrong, listen to your heartbeat and respiration*'. The men's group

**Table 19: Criteria identified for assessing the quality of health-service providers (by gender and age)**

| Quality criteria | Respondents | | | |
| --- | --- | --- | --- | --- |
| | Men | Women | Boys | Girls |
| Cure | * | * | | * |
| Cost | * | * | * | |
| Waiting time | * | * | * | * |
| Waiting place in health facility | * | | | |
| Waiting place outside facility | * | | | |
| 24-hour service | * | * | | |
| Distance | | * | | * |
| Trained medical staff | * | * | * | * |
| Staff attitude | * | * | * | * |
| Good examination | | | | * |
| Availability of medicine | | * | * | * |
| Beds available | | * | * | |
| Cleanliness | * | * | * | * |
| Cleanliness (outside/buildings) | * | | | * |
| Latrine | * | | | * |
| Equipped with medical equipment | | | * | |
| Lab facility available | | * | | * |

(Source: PRA focus-group discussions)

scored the health centre and drug store highest for cures, and traditional treatment lowest. The women also scored the health centre and hospital high for cure but included holy waters, other traditional treatments, and the TBAs among those with a high score for cure. The most costly service, and that with the least chance of a cure, women said, was that provided by illegal abortionists. They also thought drug stores were too costly. Men tend to use the drug stores and the health centre more, while women tend to go to traditional healers and the holy waters more. The reasons are a combination of access to cash, cost, distance, waiting time, and expectation of a cure.

# Education

In the adult focus groups there was a strong appreciation of the value of education, and for both girls and boys. In the past it was not as strongly appreciated that girls should go to school, but things have changed. Some women were keen that education should improve girls' opportunities and status, and mothers did not want their girls to live such a tough life as theirs. Education was broadly linked to access to employment and to the ability to look after one's family, including the parents in their old age.

However, in the household survey, where 70% of the respondents were women, as many as 33% of respondents from worst-off households thought there were no advantages to educating boys, and 43% no advantages to educating girls. All better-off households believed in the benefit of educating both girls and boys. Boys and girls thought that education could liberate the community from poverty (boys) and help them to teach their own children (girls). Both believed education would help them in their jobs in the future, but boys said that there was a need for skills training in addition to schooling to make them employable.

## Level of education in the community

Levels of education among parents and appreciation of the value of education for their offspring are connected. There were higher levels of illiteracy in the worst-off households than in the better-off, with 41% of the male heads of household and 22% of the female heads of household illiterate in the worst-off group, while in the better-off households 75% had completed Grades 9-12.

It was interesting that a higher percentage of women household-heads were literate (30% of worst-off households interviewed), than men household-heads. This may be connected to the literacy campaign during Mengistu's period, when many women and children took advantage of literacy classes in the Kebele.

## Availability of primary schooling

The only schools in the Kebele are fee-paying private schools attended by children from marginally better-off households within and outside the Kebele. The worst-off households cannot afford to send their children to these schools and have to send them to government schools outside the Kebele. The schools most used by children in this community are Edget Behbret (a government school outside the Kebele), Felege Yordanos (a private fee-paying school), and Walya community school (also fee-paying). For many households the nearest government schools are too far away. Women expressed concern for their children of primary-school age walking through the highly congested area and in the traffic. Hence most of the worst-off and medium households in the Kebele do not send their children to school.

## Children in school

The Zone 2 Education Office said that very few children in Kebele 24 actually go to school. There is no government school in the Kebele. They agreed that the government schools in the neighbouring Kebele were too far away, and added that they are also oversubscribed. In Woreda 21 as a whole there are not enough school places to accommodate all children of primary-school age.

The household survey showed that out of 59 children in the worst-off households interviewed, 41% were not in school. Although the number of years in school varied, both adult focus groups reported that boys stayed longer in school on average than girls.

For children in school, particular difficulties were reported; those reporting them included the teachers. Poverty was increasing and demonstrating itself in children's poor diet. Children reported being hungry in school and lacking concentration. Girls in particular have heavy domestic and income-earning workloads, which interfere with their performance in school and ability to fulfil homework assignments. Boys from the poorest families have difficulties because they have to work, in daily labour, hawking, or shoe-shining to supplement the family income, in addition to their school work; sometimes the household's increased need for their labour is a reason for leaving school.

Older boys are disruptive, and discipline is a major problem. The Kebele said that most of the boys taking drugs, alcohol, and tobacco are from better-off families. Those from the poorest households are busy earning money for the family.

## Reasons for not attending school, and affordability

The main reasons for not attending school are low incomes, and the cost of sending all children to school. The cost, even in government schools where parents have to pay a maximum of 10.00 Birr (US$ 1.28) as a registration fee, is prohibitive. This is also because children in primary school in Addis have to wear uniforms at a cost of Birr 50.00 – 60.00 (US$6.40 – 7.69), or one month's income. Parents in the focus groups include food, clothing, exercise books, and the cost of health care in the cost of sending a child to school. Sending one child is expensive enough; it is hard to send four–eight children to school. Education-service providers agreed that education was too expensive for the poorest households, who are in the majority in a Kebele like Cherkos.

In Kebele 24 another main reason for non-attendance is the fact that there is no government school in the Kebele. It is considered by mothers to be too distant, dangerous, and congested for children to walk to the other Kebele school. Children would also have to cross busy roads.

The unemployment or death of a parent, or serious illness in the family, affects income sufficiently for a family to withdraw one or more children from school.

Because of hunger, child-labour obligations, and the stress of poverty and living in such a congested and poor environment 'not conducive to learning', children, in particular girls, do not meet the required educational standards school. One of the most common reasons for leaving is failing a repeat year. Children are not allowed to sit an exam for a third time. Some children attend school when there is enough money, and leave school to find work when household income is too low. This also affects performance and their ability to pass exams and stay in school.

Some children and adults reported that for male adolescents in particular the attractions of street life are greater than school, and they refuse to go. Parents cannot control them. There were reports of young girls who became pregnant and left school, some becoming prostitutes, attracted by the allure of high incomes as sex workers. On the other hand, other girls suffer the fear of being raped, accosted, or abused by hooligans on the way to school; this affects their performance and attendance.

Some families simply do not understand the value of education and do not send their children to school. Others cannot manage to look after, control, and guide their children because of their long working day. The boys' group said that they wished they could have more support and guidance from their parents, the community, and the government.

## Quality of existing schools

While it is true that many children do not go to school because of low incomes and the household's demands on their labour time, it is also true that there are not enough schools to accommodate all children of primary-school age anyway. At the same time, the existing schools, even private ones, are run down and lack basic materials and facilities. The state of some buildings ranges from inadequate to being hazardous to the health of the children. None of the schools had adequate sports facilities. Some classrooms in Walya are built with sheets of iron, and have up to 105 students in a class. In all schools there was a lack of desks and chairs, even for the teachers. Average class size in one private school was between 60 and 80 children. In government schools the teacher:pupil ratio sometimes reaches 1:120. None of the schools has adequate teaching materials, and in all schools children have to share textbooks. In the private schools it was reported that one book is shared between three or four children; in the government schools it can be as high as one book to six children. The Zone 2 Education Office also regretted that there was a lack of teachers' guidebooks in some grades, which certainly affected the teaching standards.

Teachers, even in the fee-paying schools, said that children come to school hungry, which affects the quality of education and their performance. None of the schools provides any food during the day. In addition girls, in particular, complained about the insanitary conditions and the lack of toilets in schools, and all were concerned about the lack or shortage of water in school compounds.

Teachers said that there was a lack of qualified teachers, and that some teachers do not even meet the criteria specified by the new education and training policy. Parents and children also noted the poor quality of teaching. In addition, the new self-contained teaching policy was proving problematic for teachers. They are not trained to teach all subjects from Grades 1 to 4, but this is now expected of them.

Teachers are motivated, but the poor conditions, low salaries, lack of teaching materials, and the favouritism that affects access to training are counter-productive. Teachers are finding it increasingly difficult to teach unruly young boys in particular. Some said that it was distressing to teach children who are obviously suffering from poverty and hunger and who had a long day of both school and work outside school hours.

Of course, in terms of quality, examination results are important to parents, but in the context of the circumstances and needs discussed above this issue was lower down the list of quality criteria.

Felege Yordanos has a good reputation for examination results; however, it was the most expensive school in the area. Overall, people thought that the quality of education in the area had deteriorated, largely because of discipline problems, particularly hooliganism and drinking, and because of the deteriorating quality of the teachers.

## Conclusions

### Health services

The focus groups made many recommendations, summarised in Table 20, to improve the health services.

*Access, affordability, and quality*
The following supply-side factors were mentioned by focus groups.

- A lack of sufficient health-care facilities in the community.
- A shortage of appropriately qualified staff.
- A lack of basic equipment.

## Table 20: Focus-group recommendations for improvements to health services

|  | Source | | | |
|  | Men's Group | Women's Group | Boys' Group | Girls' Group |
| --- | --- | --- | --- | --- |
| Build health centres or clinics in the Kebele. | * | * | * | * |
| Improve efficiency and quality of the service. | * |  |  |  |
| Employment opportunities to earn money & improve nutritional and health status. |  | * | * |  |
| Food for work for the youth – e.g. growing vegetables – with nutritional benefits. |  |  |  | * |
| Improve environmental sanitation. |  |  | * |  |
| Equip existing clinics with medical instruments and materials. |  |  | * |  |
| Improve quality and quantity of medicine. |  | * |  |  |
| Establish new public pharmacies like the Red Cross. |  |  | * |  |
| Train traditional healers to minimise the harm they can cause through lack of awareness. |  |  | * |  |
| Government training on sterile blades and needles for government and private health centres, traditional practitioners, and the community. |  |  |  | * |
| Means to borrow money for treatment. |  | * |  |  |
| Government should help the poor in the community. |  | * |  |  |
| Government should control addictive plants. |  |  | * |  |
| Guidance and counselling for the youth. |  |  | * | * |

- A shortage of sufficient quantities of good-quality, most frequently needed medication.
- A lack of funds for health education and reproductive-health education in the community, targeted at different gender/age and occupational groups.
- A lack of investment in improving water, sanitation, housing and feeder roads; improvements in environmental health would contribute to improved overall health status in the community.
- The private clinics clearly provide an important service and are close to the community; training, particularly in reproductive health and environmental sanitation, should be extended to private practitioners as well as traditional practitioners.
- A lack of training and support for traditional practitioners, particularly TBAs and traditional physiotherapists, who used to play an important role as community health workers.
- Until three years ago people used to go to drug stores for diagnosis and medication; now drug stores are not allowed to diagnose under new regulations. A procedure is needed for selection of pharmacies, and quality control, to enable drug stores to provide diagnostic and curative services for the most common diseases. Controls on the origins, expiry dates, and quantity of drugs to be taken should be in place. Drug stores are in the community and may be the only source of medical advice close to hand.

**Funding**: The community is not in a position to contribute cash to the World Bank Social Rehabilitation and Development Fund. At least 70% of the community are classified as 'worst-off', which means low incomes, 90% of income spent on food, overcrowded housing, and family sizes of at least 10 people. The Kebele has had a series of NGO, multilateral, and bilateral donors visiting and discussing programmes, with no outcome. The population is increasing, not through inward migration but through growing families. There is no investment in the area, and the situation is appalling. The Kebele is very disillusioned by development organisations which come and go, take their time discussing 'and taking photos', and then do nothing.

There must be alternatives to cash-contribution deals, which could include labour and food for work for different age and gender groups in the community.

**Demand-side problems:** The difference between city life and the rural sites is that in Addis all the basic needs have to be paid for every month: rent, electricity, water, food, and firewood/kerosene to cook and heat the house. This puts an enormous strain on the poorest households.

- Government health-service providers and private clinics and drug stores said that only with improvement in the people's economic status would their health improve.
- Health care, both preventative and curative, is unaffordable for the majority – staying healthy is unaffordable.
- Increased incomes would improve nutrition and increase access to government health services and treatment at private clinics.
- The above recommendations, linked to improvements in sanitation, incomes, and reproductive health, would improve the quality of life, increase access to better nutrition, and reduce the incidence of disease.
- Low incomes and labour-intensive work for small returns mean that there is barely enough money to feed the family, still less to contemplate paying for health services and education for four to eight children.
- Labour-intensive domestic and income-generation activities reduce the time available to go to health facilities. Women in particular wait until their condition is serious.
- Unemployment, low incomes, and lack of opportunities for the young in particular have resulted in a deterioration in the social fabric, an increase in juvenile delinquency, and insecurity in the streets with street violence and abuse, rape, early pregnancies, and girls taking up street trade ('streetism').
- All focus groups linked improved health and nutrition to employment, incomes, and/or food-for-work programmes. Young girls in particular wanted employment for male youth, who were described as being disturbed in their minds and disruptive in the community.
- Sexual promiscuity, early pregnancy, and large family sizes are a burden on low-income households, put pressure on the housing situation, and increase the spread of STDs and HIV/AIDS. Reproductive-health education in the community must be a priority.

### Gendered division of labour and responsibilities

Women in the worst-off households suffer a particularly heavy burden of responsibility to find the cash to feed the family each day. They have a long working day, including carrying heavy loads in domestic and income-earning activities. Their reproductive-health status is poor and characterised by early pregnancy, high fertility rates, and deliveries at home, a high incidence of anaemia, indicative of a poor diet, and postnatal heavy bleeding, with little or no medical assistance, all in the context of the abysmal sanitary conditions.

- Men suffer unemployment, are reduced to occasional daily labour jobs at low incomes, and are said to turn to alcohol. A man's contribution to household income, according to focus-group participants, makes a significant difference to the welfare of the family. Men need to be re-engaged with family life.
- Investment in employment creation for both women and men would be invaluable.
- Investment in water points and sanitation would reduce women's and girls' workloads.
- Programmes to address alcoholism, drug addiction, and tobacco consumption would release some cash for food in the household, and reduce multiple, high-risk sexual relations and improve men's health status.
- Food-for-work programmes are needed in water, sanitation, road building, etc., to involve the youth (both male and female), together with training in masonry, building, plumbing, etc., for future employment.

## Education

The recommendations made by women and men to improve the accessibility and quality of education are summarised in Table 21.

**Access to education:** In the household survey the broad recommendations to improve access to education included adequate food; adequate clothing; availability of sufficient income; well-equipped schools, sufficient learning materials and good teachers; free education; and convenient location. These conditions for improvement are almost identical to those mentioned by the girls' youth group, and many are included in the recommendations from the PRA.

It is absolutely clear that the cost of education does not consist solely of registration fees. The cost of education is the cost of keeping a child fed and healthy and providing him/her with a uniform and exercise books and pens. It is also the cost of replacing the money normally earned by the child in school. It is the opportunity-cost

## Table 21: Focus-group recommendations for improvements to education services

| Recommendations | W | M |
|---|---|---|
| Improve the security situation in the area as a whole (crime). | * | * |
| Improve security for both boys and girls. | * | |
| Take action to reduce harassment of girls. | | * |
| Clean up the school environment, inc. toilets and water supply. | * | * |
| Need properly constructed classrooms. | * | |
| Establish sufficient good schools (quantity and quality); | * | * |
| and make them free. | * | |
| Have capable teachers; | | * |
| more and better trained teachers. | * | |
| Follow up families, monitor children's performance. | | * |
| Create good contact with the teachers. | | * |
| Government should discuss with us to improve schooling. | * | |
| Government should provide enough books & teaching materials; | * | |
| should sell exercise books, pens and pencils at production price on school premises. | * | |
| Community has to cooperate with PTA, school, and government to improve schools and control children. | * | |
| *'About school uniform, it's a good idea, but we can't afford to pay for it.'* | * | |
| Need sports fields/facilities. | * | |

of women's lost income if they have to stay at home and do the domestic tasks normally done by their daughters while they are trading or employed in daily labour. These costs in the poorest households have to be multiplied by four to eight children.

Education is not affordable. Nor is it available, since there are not enough school places and not enough books and desks and chairs.

**Quality of education:** service providers made the following recommendations to improve the quality of education.

- Children should not be hungry.
- Teachers' salaries should be improved.
- Well-trained teachers must be assigned to schools. Political appointees who have no interest in teaching and who are academically and pedagogically incompetent should not be posted as teachers.

- Adequate instructional materials, facilities, and equipment must be made available.
- In the case of Felege Yordanos: either change the market-place or demolish the existing school and have it rebuilt elsewhere.
- Additional classrooms should be constructed, particularly at Edget Behbret School.
- Reasonably wide playgrounds and sports equipment should be provided.
- All of the above cannot be realised by individual efforts nor by the communities themselves. The view of the educational establishment is that the government has to be involved by way of providing land, trained teachers, and ample instructional materials and facilities.

# Appendix 4
# Case study 2: Yegurassa and Andaje, Delanta Dawunt, North Wollo

The research site in Peasant Association (PA) 05 was selected by the Oxfam Regional Office in Delanta. It was chosen because Oxfam does not have a regular commitment to the PA, and no participatory research had been conducted with this community. Although only 15km from Wogel Tena, the capital of Delanta Dawunt woreda, the site was a one hour's drive away over rough terrain. The team decided to select two neighbouring villages, Yegurassa and Andaja, within 30 minutes' walk of each other. This facilitated logistics during the household interviews and service-providers' phase. There were about 70–80 households in each village. The school and church were located in a third village, Wokote, about 30 minutes' walk from Yegurassa.

## Poverty, nutrition, and livelihoods

### Poverty

During the mapping, the women and men involved ranked 60 households from the two villages (about 40% of the population) according to their own poverty criteria. They dismissed the notion of 'poor', 'medium', and 'better-off' categories. Instead, they ranked the households: most vulnerable (13% of households), very poor (80%), and better-off (7%). Well-being is ranked according to livestock ownership, including horses and donkeys. Women-headed households are also ranked in this way. Although livestock are viewed as a household asset, it is the men who sell the livestock and control the income from the sale. Livestock ownership is also used by officials to means-test the population. A household with sufficient livestock can gain access to agricultural credit, will not be issued with an exemption paper for health care, and will not receive food aid.

However, due to persistent harvest failures over the past seven years, most households 'have nothing'. Gradually, people who were better-off have become as poor as those categorised as 'very poor', with only one cow and horse, or two sheep, because they have sold their animals to

buy food. The 'most vulnerable' are mostly households where there are no animals at all, one or more income-earners (men or women) are seriously ill, or where the man has died or left to the lowlands, reducing the household's potential daily income.

### Nutrition

Without harvests there is no food. Over 90% of income in the most vulnerable and very poor households is used to buy food. Average income in 70% of these households is less than 50.00 Birr per month ($US6.40); in another 26%, average income is below 100.00 birr per month. As a last resort, animals are sold. The population of PA 05 has no choice but to fall back on very basic means of survival, using dung, straw, trees, and their own physical strength to survive.

A crucial feature is that among an estimated 93% of the population in the two villages researched, more or less 60% eat only twice a day. At least one meal, if not both, is likely to be very insubstantial. Almost one-third eat only once a day, and some say that is just a cup of coffee to keep them going. Almost 50% of women in the most vulnerable group eat only once a day. We know that some do not eat at all.

There is minimal outside support or intervention. The community remembers the 1980s, when the Derg's government provided food and clothes when they had nothing. The Ministry of Agriculture's woreda office is involved in development activities, some of which are co-ordinated and funded through the Integrated Food Security Project, a project funded by the European Union and overseen by Oxfam. Its activities include soil and water conservation; pond construction (food for work in Yegurassa Gote); capacity-building for farmers; horticulture; private nurseries; provision of tools and pesticides and sprays to the woreda agricultural office; and, via the woreda administrative office, roads construction (also a food-for-work programme).

However, given the gravity of the current situation, the lack of tree cover, the lack of water for agriculture or home consumption, and the lack of feed for livestock, visible externally driven development activity in Yegurassa, Andaja, and Wokote villages is minimal. The project is facilitated through MoA development agents, who are responsible for up to 800 households (about eight Gotes). Under existing conditions, this is like sifting sand in the wilderness.

In many families about 90% of income is spent on food, and on totally inadequate amounts at that. Families cope by living from hand to mouth (*'ke idge waddey aff'*). There were strong indicators that men, women, and children are suffering from malnutrition. Men said that women and children suffer more. We heard reports of a high incidence of miscarriage attributed to malnutrition (men's group and TBAs reporting). Children complain of hunger and stomach pains, and eat one or two small meals a day (women's group and children's groups reporting). Many children go to school without breakfast or with very little. Most people are eating 'kolo. Some families are eating guaya, which is a plant that can be *'eaten like njera or fried. When we eat it hot, it breaks us.'* It is a drought-resistant plant, known to cause permanent lameness: *'He became lame because he ate guaya, but we eat it all the same because of lack of alternatives'* (men's group). Some parents reported drinking coffee and going the whole day with nothing – giving what little grain there was to the children.

They said they *'appeal to the Kebele officials for assistance to get grain every month in exchange for our labour'*. Unfortunately the local food-for-work programme in Yegurassa had not supplied any food 'payment' in the past four months. It was finally distributed during the research week (February 1999), a few days before the major 'Kebre Ba'al religious festival. The grain was used up to prepare for the visitors coming from surrounding villages to the festival.

The men said that there was little left to do but pray. While the research was going on, they were waiting every day for the rain to come, so they could plant seeds: *'God is almighty, he saves us. Our coping strategy depends upon God. We go to church and pray.'* The rain never came.

### Water and sanitation

The women collect water from local springs, of which three were highlighted in the mapping: Gurassa Tana, Tiburay spring in Andaja village, and Ambo spring, which is far away. One of the main problems raised by the focus groups was a shortage of water, and a need for clean water. One woman said: *'Why do you think the flies are all around us, we are dirty.'* One girl explained: *'I can't wash because it's too cold and my hands are already sore from the cold.'* Her hands were ingrained with dirt, rough and sore. And people have no clothes to change into when they have washed. It is a highland climate, and the wind is cold. Skin problems and scabies are common complaints, attributed to hunger and sanitation. Again, there is very little being done about the water situation in PA 05. A pond is being dug in Yegurassa as part of a food-for-work programme. It was extraordinary to find people (mostly men and boys) digging at the hard rock, despite not having received their monthly food payment for four months. This would be an indication of dire need, even if there were no others.

There are no latrines or waste-disposal facilities. People use the open countryside. The country is open and clean, and there are no visible signs of human waste or other rubbish. However, most people are dirty and unwashed. The high incidence of diarrhoea was attributed by men and women to dirty water and flies. The youth focus groups told us that at school they are told about the benefits of washing and staying clean. One mother said: *'They teach her that she should wash with soap and water.'* She thought this was very good; but, asked whether she could buy soap, the woman laughed: *'What do you think? Of course not!'*

A doctor at the health centre attributed the high incidence of diseases to *'poverty, a low level of awareness of health, problem of safe water, even the tap water is contaminated (in the town), poor personal hygiene and poor environmental sanitation'*. The woreda has a sanitation officer, but the department is understaffed and under-resourced. According to health-centre staff, there are no funds at all for environmental sanitation work, particularly for work in schools and prisons. The staff undertake this work without a budget.

### Livelihoods

*'The people have difficulties to find their earning unless they exchange something: goat, sheep, cow dung, firewood.'*

With the main livelihood base (livestock and crop production) eroded, men and women, with a significant contribution from their children, have shifted to daily, labour-intensive activities, with minimal returns. Even those who still have some livestock *'are even worse off, because they have to worry about their feed'* (women's group). The selling price for cattle has dropped by 65%. The men said, '*We get our food by purchasing, and the money comes from selling wood, grass, cow dung, casual labour working as livestock tending*', the latter largely by girls and boys, some as young as four and five years old.

Now, according to the household survey, 29% of men and 12% of women are engaged in food-for-work or daily labour activities. Another 57% of men were involved in collecting, transporting, and selling items such as firewood and grass (large bales of which are used for thatching roofs). In a third of the households interviewed, women also collect, transport, and sell firewood, often as one of several income-earning activities. Men, women, and children go down the steep slopes of the gorge and cut firewood to carry and sell in the market (one day's work = 3.00 birr). It is a hazardous occupation, and there are fatal accidents.

Collecting and selling cow dung for fuel has become a key source of daily income, with 71% of women reporting it (two days' work = 2.00 birr ($US 0.26) for a large basketful). This used to be one of women's income-earning activities to bridge food shortages until a harvest, but now it appears to have become a more regular main source of income for many households. Women also collect, transport, and weave sheep's wool, 38% of women, all from the most vulnerable or very poor households, reporting it (10 balls of wool: eight days' work = 2.00 – 3.00 birr); and they weave baskets for sale, 25% of women from all poverty categories reporting it.

Some men cut and strip young eucalyptus saplings to sell in the market and share the returns. They are conscious of the fact that they are in effect destroying the environment to survive: '*We are all struggling selling wood, dung and wool. We are now tired and the eucalyptus is also lost*', but they have no choice.

The men's focus group discussed the implications of drought and the Global 2000 credit scheme. '*We get fertilisers and improved seeds on a credit basis. After the crops were destroyed, we were forced to pay the credit. We sell our animals and goods, which takes us into more poverty. Those who could not pay are taken to prison, which means more worse situation than three years ago.*' A TBA said, '*The credit scheme is provided without the appropriate education. We are being imprisoned, as we cannot afford to pay on time. Because of the drought people cannot keep their promises.*'

A small but ever-increasing number of men migrate to the lowlands in search of work. Some young girls are also sent to the lowlands to do bar work. It is not without risks: '*Last month there were five deaths. All five had gone to the lowlands in search of jobs but came back with yellow malaria and died. There are another ten or more who have returned from the lowlands sick and are in bed waiting to die,*' a TTBA told us. In a society where it is important to have a man who can bring in additional income and represent the family in public decisions and claim access to resources, women left behind with children can become even worse off. When income diminishes and women's burden increases, the need to increase the contribution of children's labour arises and often results in their leaving school. It is an essential survival strategy for the family as a whole. One girl said: '*If our fathers could grow crops, we could go to school full-time.*'

### Child labour

Girls' and boys' labour – looking after animals, collecting and selling firewood (boys and girls), collecting dung for the market (girls), and domestic work (girls) – is central to daily life. The drought and consequent reduced agricultural activity has reduced the need for boys' labour in agriculture. Boys instead have to contribute their labour to daily income-earning activities such as collecting firewood. The heaviest burden is, however, still borne by girls, although boys' labour time also interferes with their school attendance.

# Health

The main health problems identified by men were typhoid fever, diarrhoea, mogne bagegne, and pregnancy and associated problems; by women: mogne bagegne, scabies, headache and nausea, rheumatic pains, ear aches (from insect in the ear), and heavy menstrual bleeding. The main health problems suffered by youth and children, as identified by girls, were diarrhoea, scabies, and accidents (e.g. when collecting firewood); by boys: typhoid fever, mogne bagegne, scabies, and abdominal pains. The traditional healers and the health centre identified more or less the same main health problems. The traditional healers were concerned by the extent of illness in the community and attributed it very much to poverty and hunger. They said that people come with stomach problems when they eat something after being hungry for too long. Women said '*Many people die because they cannot afford health treatment.*'

## Reproductive health

Harmful traditional practices such as female and male circumcision (genital mutilation) are still widely practised. According to all focus groups and education-service providers interviewed, early marriage was one of the main reasons why girls leave school. Early pregnancy is common.

In none of the households interviewed did women go to the health centre to give birth; 89% gave birth at home, 4% at a TBA's, and 7% at a relative's. The health centre in Wogel Tena is a three-hour walk away. Women and girls experiencing obstructed birth or other irregularities are likely to die, according to the health-centre doctor. The hospital in Dessie is a four-hour drive away from Wogel Tena, and few can afford the transport.

All focus groups were aware of HIV/AIDS and said that young people were dying from it.

## Access to health-service providers

There is one health centre in Wogel Tena, a three-hour walk from the site. The doctor: population ratio is 1:161,966. Most households use traditional healers or go to holy waters at the church in Wokote. They largely cannot afford the government health services, which are too far away. Very few have access to an exemption paper: *'At present the PA doesn't provide us with a paper, because we are all poor and are all asking for the paper'* (women's group). The PA leaders confirmed that *'the woreda office has told the PA that anyone with livestock, even one hen, is not eligible for an exemption paper, so they [the PA] are unable to issue exemption papers to most of the people. People cannot afford the fees at the health centre, so they don't go.'* The PA leaders had gone to the woreda health office explaining the situation in January (Tir). They had had no reply. They know that the woreda has no budget.

The health centre is under-resourced. Seventy-five per cent of its patients are 'free', and most come from the town of Wogel Tena. The doctor at the health centre said: *'Most cannot afford, the situation has deteriorated as they have become poorer and poorer.'* Ninety-three per cent of households interviewed said health services were *'unaffordable'*. Of the rural population, it is mostly men who come to the health centre. The health centre said that women and children do not come for treatment until they are seriously ill; they go to holy waters first, believing they can find cures, especially for particular diseases like scabies. The girls' group also said that better-off people were favoured, so they did not like the health centre: *'They do not care for weaker people.'*

When in need, women and men sell assets or borrow or ask neighbours for help in order to cover health costs. Men, and women heads of household, rent out their land in exchange for cash or crops in order to cover costs. However, for better-off farmers (mostly men), the drought has reduced the attractiveness of renting land. Some men leave the area in search of work as casual labourers, with the intention of sending money to pay for health costs.

Families 'cope' with education costs and health care during bad times by simply withdrawing their children from school, and staying at home without treatment, respectively. They say that many are dying as a result. Some of the traditional healers are providing treatment free of charge, because people cannot pay.

Finally, the MCH outreach programme stopped eight months ago, when UNICEF's programme came to an end. Children born in the past eight months did not even have one dose of antigens. There is little chance that infants under one year will complete their full doses.

# Education

There is one elementary school in Wokote: Tana Elementary School, Grades 1–6. To complete primary education (Grades 7–8), children have to walk for three hours to the Wogel Tena Elementary School. Consequently very few children complete school, and most who do are boys. The women said that girls are in danger of becoming pregnant if they go to the town.

There is hunger and disease, and clothing is inadequate. An estimated 60% of the children in the community do not attend school. In addition, among those who attend, absenteeism was a major problem highlighted by Wokote teachers. Boys miss one day per week on average, and girls two days per week, because of demands on their labour. Class sizes vary enormously. In Wokote Grade 1 is a group of over 253. The number drops off to 14 in Grade 6. In the woreda as a whole, attendance numbers drop from 4739 students in Grade 1 to 427 in Grade 8. For the past three years the woreda education office has been pursuing a policy of increasing school enrolment. Parents said they were *'forced'* to send their children to school. In the woreda as a whole, 58% of primary-school children are boys and 42% girls. The boys' group said they thought that more girls should attend school. A major reason for girls' low attendance was domestic work and early marriage.

The woreda education office confirmed what the community told us: '*Large proportions of children, and about more than half of girls, do not attend school. The reasons are poverty and repeated famine, early marriage, and parents' unwillingness to send children to school.*'

Although in the focus groups both women and men were in favour of educating both boys and girls, 57% of very poor households interviewed did not see the value of educating girls, and 14% did not see the value of educating boys. In the households interviewed, 70% of adults were illiterate themselves. The men's group, however, said that there had been a change in attitudes: '*Before a few years parents wanted their boys to work in agriculture and girls to work at home with their mothers. Now they have understood the value of education for both boys and girls. But poverty arising from natural calamity since 1991 is now the obstacle.*' Despite the great optimism vested in the value of education, the men's group expressed a very serious doubt: '*There is also dissatisfaction among parents, because those who have completed grade 12 from our community could not get jobs, or continue their education beyond grade 12.*'

More or less 70% of the local population earn less than 50.00 Birr ($US6.4) per month; 96% earn less than 100.00 Birr ($12.80) per month. In these families, 75–92% of income is spent on food. Children are too hungry to go to school and have inadequate clothing. In theory schooling is free, but parents included food, clothes, and exercise books in the cost of schooling. They cannot afford these items. The Education Office in Wogel Tena is fully aware of the situation, and said that education was '*too expensive, especially for poor people*'.

The schools lack textbooks (one book to eight pupils), chairs, desks, water, toilets, and teaching materials. The buildings require substantial maintenance work, and there are no sports or recreational facilities. There is a budget of 300.00 Birr per year for medicines for the 24 schools in the woreda. The schools receive teachers' salaries and very little else. They grow grass and some vegetables to sell towards their income. Basically, the schools are under-resourced, and there is no external funding to improve the situation even marginally.

In Wokote there are no women teachers or staff. Women from the community were clearly less informed about the school than men are. There were no women in the school committee. All education-service providers said that boys do better than girls in school, and put this down to early marriage and the labour demands made on girls. They also said that girls were not as interested as boys in education, and that parents do not encourage them enough. The girls also said that they have problems when menstruating. They miss school and cannot explain the reason to the male teachers. All told, girls have particular problems which are not managed, and they themselves feel discriminated against. Boys attending the Wogel Tena primary school (Grades 7–8), on the other hand, feel that boys from the urban areas are favoured by the teachers, and they are discriminated against.

The men's group thought that their school in Wokote had more difficulties than the school in Wogel Tena, because it is physically so far from the woreda authorities in town. They believed that problems could be dealt with more easily by schools in town. The research, however, shows that both rural and urban schools have very similar problems. They both need maintenance, have inadequate playing facilities, no water or toilets, and lack teaching materials, textbooks, desks, and chairs, and the classrooms are overcrowded. Yet there are some rural/urban differences. The repetition rate in Wogel Tena is lower, and children in rural Wokote are on average two years behind their peers in the town.

## Conclusions and recommendations

'*If we get clothing, food and adequate medical care, we would be most comfortable*' (women's focus group). The following section lists aspirations expressed by the community, disaggregated by gender and generation.

### Women's aspirations and recommendations

*Livelihoods*

- Make better roads for vehicles to pass.
- Establish a new market.
- Build a grinding mill near the school.
- Deal with cattle diseases.
- NGOs should give us skills to be productive.
- Establish food-for-work programmes.
- Hopes: to harvest barley as they used to before.

*Nutrition*

- Provision of food rationing until the situation improves.

*Water and sanitation*

- Install tap water near the primary school.

*Health*

- Have a health station located near the school in Wokote.
- Have clothing, food, and adequate medical care.
- Free treatment, especially for women and children.
- Medicines: *'The government is what we have next to God'.*
- *'We want the government to realise that even if we have a health centre with equipment, we are dying of illness.'*

*Education*

- Establish a school for Grades 7-8 near the existing primary school.
- Provide free exercise books and pens..

## Men's aspirations and recommendations

*Livelihoods*

- Construct a road to Wogel Tena (*'We have already contributed 5.00 Birr'*).
- Establish a system of irrigation to make farming possible.
- Establish provision of free seeds and fertiliser.
- Establish food for work programmes.

*Nutrition*

- Establish provision of food rationing until the situation improves.

*Water and sanitation*

- Solve the shortage of water problem (*'Oxfam already been helping with water'*).
- Install tap water near the primary school.
- *'We need clothes and soap.'*

*Health*

- NGOs to open clinics in nearby villages.
- Construct a clinic in the area with help from the community.
- Have a health station located near the school in Wokote.
- Establish provision of free treatment.

*Education*

- Establish a school for Grades 7–8 near the existing primary school.
- Need a government policy to assist and support children from very poor households.

- Provide free exercise books and pens.
- Help to meet needs for clothing food and stationery.
- School should farm land with assistance from local NGOs and provide free lunch to children from vulnerable and very poor households.

## Girls' aspirations and recommendations

*Livelihoods*

- Food-for-work programmes.

*Health and sanitation*

- Stop medicines being sold off by the health centre (to private pharmacies).
- Need medication to cure scabies.
- The government should stop favouring the people who can pay.
- *'We don't need a new health centre, we want the services at the existing one improved.'*
- Need adult education at the Kebele for our parents in birth spacing, preparing nutritious food, and clean preparation of food, personal and house hygiene.

*Education*

- Enough clothes.
- Enough grain.
- Rain and harvests, *'so we would go to school instead of collecting dung and firewood to sell'*.
- Grinding mills *'so that children don't have to grind'*.
- Domestic servants *'so we would not have to do domestic work and we could go to school'*.

## Boys' aspirations and recommendations

*Health*

- Have a health station located nearby, preferably well equipped.
- Have a health centre with qualified staff.
- Medicines
- To have research conducted into existing traditional medicines, their application and effectiveness, and to make them available to the public.
- Need adult education on circumcision and family planning for parents.
- Need lessons in literacy centres and to strengthen the health-education service at the health centre.

*Education*

- Increase the number of girls attending school.
- Teachers should care about all students.
- Provide water and sanitation in school.
- Improved quality of teaching.
- Provision of schools nearby.
- Remove poverty, to increase attendance.
- Provide food and health care to increase attendance.
- Clergymen ('debtera') should be trained to stop their evil practices on some students.

### What could the community do?

People are painfully conscious of their poverty and suffering. Women talked about men who have no clothing in which to go out and do daily work, and who have no energy: *'Due to frost their feet are not able to move, some of them sit and die.'* Men talked about women's problems: *'Due to drought effect, our women are malnourished and give birth to unhealthy children.'* The only thing the community can do is to continue the struggle to survive. The men say that the community can do nothing more than that. The woreda education office confirmed that the community could not, for example, contribute to the costs of improving education, *'because the community is very poor'.*

## Recommendations: potential for action

Despite the very negative findings of the survey, the meeting with the PA administration demonstrated that there are key social institutions (run by men) which manage some parts of community life, and provide channels of communication to institutions outside the community. These include the church, the Kerray, and the PA (in which two out of 69 officials are women). In the Kerray and PA, household heads are members representing their families. Women are therefore members only if they are widows or divorced. The fact that men dominate all institutions is traditional, rather than rational, given the degree to which men in the focus group openly recognised women's contribution and problems.

Future initiatives should be taken with existing social institutions, increasing the representation of all gender and age interests and needs.

## Tackling contributors to poverty and gender inequities

In theory, if the contributors to poverty and lack of purchasing power (in an economy which requires cash to pay for basic needs and services) are tackled, then women and men could better access health services for themselves and their children. They could also cover the basic requirements necessary to enable their children to attend school. The contributors to poverty include three broad domains: *natural*; *external*: international, government, and NGO policy and planning; and *internal*: cultural factors.

### The 'natural' domain

The hostile weather conditions over the past seven years have contributed to repeated lost harvests. As a result, traditional share-cropping relations have broken down, and there is no food and no income from the sale of crops. In addition, livestock ownership has been depleted, and traditional shareholding arrangements have broken down. Because of the complete dependency of these highland communities on crop production and livestock, women and men have few resources to fall back on.

It is not possible to influence nature, but it is possible to develop support strategies, combined with a strengthening of women's and men's capacity to cope under these circumstances. This requires a substantial increase in financial and human resources. At the moment, however, certain government initiatives, such as the agricultural credit programme, exacerbate the situation, and threaten individual households' very survival. Equally, there is a general lack of external intervention to strengthen women's and men's resolve and ability to manage under such adverse conditions.

### External: international, government, and NGO policy and planning

Loss of crops and cattle, together with lack of government intervention or NGO back-up, leaves people destitute, with no means to eat, send their children to school, or treat increasing incidences of illness.

*Livelihoods and food security*

**Agricultural credit:** *'Even if the government gave seed to help us, the land could not give grain'* (women's focus group). The government has provided grain seed on credit, the repayment of

**Table 22: Institutions in the community with potential for action**

| Institution | Function | Management | Membership |
|---|---|---|---|
| Church | Centre of life. Teaches religious instruction. Blesses the fields. Cures illnesses. Settles disputes. | Church committee of priests: all men | Men and women in the community; men play a more decisive role. |
| 'Kerray | Informal savings association for weddings, funerals, and religious festivals. One or two 'Kerray in each Gote. | Heads of households (men or women) represent the families | Men and women |
| 'Kerray Abatoch | Meets to plan very large festivals. Solves serious crime – theft or murder. Holds court and punishes culprit. Most severe punishment is banishment from Kerray = banishment from church. No links to woreda admin or courts and system of justice. | Each 'kerray has elected Elders; five of these Elders form the 'Kerray Abatoch of PA 05. | Only men, no women Elders. |
| Peasant Association | Link between community and development or local government. NGOs & government work with community through PA. Has organisational structure down to each Gote. PA is an animator and disseminator of information. | Has its own management structure. | 69 members, 2 of whom are women. |
| Service co-operative | Is dysfunctional. Was set up to sell essentials to the community. Obviously important to the community. | For the time being none, but would be elected by the community. | Probably heads of household men or women. |
| Elementary school committee | Deals with problems in the school; Animates community to improve school (fencing etc). Organises farming of school land to contribute to school funds. | School staff ; PA representatives; Community. | Men; Men; Men. |

(Source: Meeting with PA 05 Administration)

which has created more problems. The PA has sought to resolve this at the woreda agricultural office, without much success. The exertion to repay agricultural credit further exacerbates a very precarious existence for many households. Livestock, which were used as collateral, have been sold to buy food. Some men have left for the lowlands to work to repay the credit, while women and children survive on even less daily income. Through advocacy at national level with the Ministry of Agriculture, and capacity-building at woreda and PA levels, action should be taken to resolve the immediate dilemma and to develop strategies for future agricultural-

credit defaults, which are inevitable in drought-prone regions like north Wollo.

**Food aid:** *'Because of the drought the government should provide us with grain. The previous government provided clothing, blankets and since the land was not producing they settled us somewhere else.'* Both the men's and women's groups referred to the fact that the previous government had provided food aid and clothing. The methodology used in the early warning system, inter-related as it is with pre-harvest crop assessments and the Global 2000 agricultural credit initiative, potentially creates a conflict of interests for Ministry of Agriculture personnel. As a result it appears that the woreda and zone agricultural and DPPC offices cannot agree on food-aid requirement figures. The woreda office is afraid that the figures are greatly underestimated: *'In the past three to four years the people have tried to exist in different ways and now have no alternatives to assist themselves – the only alternative is to migrate south,'* said one very worried official. They estimated that 60% of PA 05 was in need of food aid (February 1999). They say that even the food-for-work and employment-generating activities cannot help the people, as the problem has been going on for too long. Any food-for-work programme should be sure to make food 'payments' each month. Men working at the pond-construction project in Yegurassa complained they had not received their food in payment for their labour for the past four months. More food-for-work initiatives should be taken to respond to needs expressed by women and men in the community. These could include water provision and road construction. In addition, men are aware of the fact that they are depleting environmental resources in order to survive. Research into appropriate tree species and tree planting should be taking place on a large scale. (For example, it is known in the community that eucalyptus drains the soil of nutrients, which is why they do not plant it along the fields.) EU funding and the Oxfam programme include these activities. However, their contributions are simply not enough.

**Veterinary services:** The PA representatives said that the MoA provides veterinary services. The women's group said that they need help to cure cattle diseases. During the cold season, and during the extreme heavy rains, they need help to resolve problems with livestock. On the basis of experience of previous re-stocking programmes, it is recommended that action should be taken to assist households to increase their livestock resources again, once appropriate conditions prevail. Gender implications of livestock ownership, and also the food-security implications, should be taken into account so that women can also benefit from any such initiative.

**Other livelihood sources:** At least 70% of the adult population in the villages interviewed were illiterate. Women in particular were looking to the NGO community to provide training opportunities to broaden livelihood options.

**Reducing domestic workloads:** Provision of accessible clean water and establishment of grinding mills would reduce the amount of time that women and girls have to spend on domestic work. This would increase the time available for schooling, and potentially increase time available for involvement in other activities – both income-earning initiatives, and, for example, work with the PA or school committee. Women's workloads impede them from going to the health centre before an illness becomes too serious.

*Health services*
The staff at the woreda department of health and personnel at the health centre are aware of the enormous health problems that the people of Delanta have to face. They state that the poor have no access to health services, that the budget for treatment is low, and that outreach services are not sustained.

**Infrastructure and transport:** The Woreda Health Department said that two clinics and five health posts have been constructed in the past five years. The main problem is a shortage of staff and resources. Only two of the new health posts are actually functioning. The staff would like to provide free basic health services through an increased number of health institutions *'at the door step of the poor'*. They also wish for government provision of additional relief drugs, supplied free, to improve curative services to the poor. The health centre desperately needs transport, in particular an ambulance, and a generator to maintain a permanent source of electricity.

**Curative and outreach services:** It is clear that the rural population does not have access to curative services. Since the UNICEF funds for vaccine and antenatal outreach services stopped, people have had no access to basic MCH services either. The reproductive-health status of women and girls is life-threateningly serious. MCH outreach services are required, as are antenatal outreach services, in conjunction with TBA training and support. The schoolteachers are potential allies in community awareness-raising on the subjects of early marriage, early pregnancy, and general sexual-health matters for boys and girls. There is a need for at least one woman teacher who can act as an advocate for girls and provide them with sexual-health education. To this end also the school and PA should be encouraged to create a gender balance on the school committee. Women are too overworked to take active community roles; this should be discussed and solutions found. If the PA administration is to be a partner in improving outreach services, increasing women's representation and action is essential. The health centre also needs an increase in supplies of the most frequently required basic medications.

**Support and training for health staff:** The existing health infrastructure in the woreda is not adequately staffed or resourced. There is no adequate budget for supervision and training, which would enable motivated health workers in the remote rural areas to perform their duties more efficiently. Both the woreda and the health-centre staff said that they had asked Oxfam GB to supply an ambulance. They wished Oxfam would have some input on the woreda health sector, as it has on the agriculture sector of the woreda. Staff at both the woreda department of health and the health centre strongly feel that the woreda health department should be able to utilise part of the income generated from service fees to fill the gaps that are not covered by the budget or by other sources such as UNICEF and IDA funds.

*Education*

**Child labour:** One of the main reasons why children do not attend school is that their labour is essential to their family's income. Girls do domestic work to enable their mothers to collect and sell cow dung and firewood. Boys who collect firewood and grasses, and girls who collect cow dung and firewood, contribute to the family income. When most incomes are as low as 50-100 Birr per month, the need is indisputable. Children will be released for school from these responsibilities when women's and men's productivity and income increase sufficiently to cover the basic costs of living. The demand on girls' labour time is greater than on boys', because of time-consuming domestic work and the burden of labour on women, which girls are expected to relieve. When domestic work is lightened, or shared beyond the female members of the household, girls will have more time to go to school and do homework.

**Cost of schooling:** Although primary education is free, parents still face unaffordable costs of items such as food, clothing, exercise books, and pens. Some children leave school because their family cannot afford to buy exercise books. Some families send only one or two children, because they cannot afford the books for all the children. Most households have a problem feeding their children, and most start the day without breakfast or with just a handful of roasted barley grains ('kolo). A solution needs to

be found, working together with women and men in the community, the school, the woreda office, and the NGO community. If the reason for non-attendance is lack of food, clothing, and exercise books, a source of subvention in the interim must be identified. If the reason is early marriage or child labour, then more complex solutions need to be discussed.

**Repairing and equipping the existing school:** The Tana Elementary School, Wokote, is the only school available for Andaja, Yegorasa, and several other neighbouring villages. It was established during the Derg period, and now the building has grown so old that it is about to fall down. The following measures are necessary: repairs to the existing school; the provision of adequate furniture – benches, chairs, and tables – for teachers and students, and sufficient textbooks for all subjects and teachers' guides; improvements to the quality of teachers, by providing in-service teacher education programme to all teachers and not to the political cadres only; the provision of clean and safe water and toilets.

**Upgrading the existing school:** The Tana Elementary School provides primary education up to Grade 6 only, two grades short of a complete primary education. It is necessary to upgrade the school to Grade 8, so that as many children as possible can finish elementary schooling.

**Constructing a new school:** The Tana Elementary School is too far away for many children, who have to walk for one and a half or nearly two hours to school. Participants in the mapping session (both women and men) recommended that a new school should be built in another Got (village), providing for Grades 1–10, and ultimately Grades 11–12.

**Internal: cultural factors**

**Early marriage, early pregnancy:** Both girls and boys said that they have sex education in school. However, 90% of respondents to the household questionnaire did not use family-planning methods. Protected sex is not widespread among adults, and is therefore unlikely to be practised by teenagers. Girls risk becoming pregnant from as early as 12 or 13, either through relationships entered voluntarily or through forced relations in early marriage arrangements. Girls are married as early as 10 years. The practice appears to be quite common and was mentioned by most focus groups, and by traditional and government providers of health and education services. Not only do early marriage and early pregnancy put an end to girls' schooling, but early pregnancy also poses a life-threatening health risk to young girls. The woreda and local elementary-school staff believe that more should be done to reverse such harmful traditional practices. According to the men's group, the school already tries to educate the community. However, the practice continues to be widespread. More needs to be done to protect young girls from early marriage and to give them choices in education and future partners.

**Female and male circumcision (genital mutilation):** All children are circumcised at a young age. Although women and girls generally did not believe that female genital mutilation was harmful, some girls knew that it could cause problems in childbirth. This was confirmed by the government health workers who were interviewed. The National Policy on Women in Ethiopia discourages both early marriage and female genital mutilation. A more intensive education and awareness-raising programme needs to be initiated with women and men, and girls and boys, and with traditional circumcisers and birth attendants in the community. The local schools and the health posts and health centre could be actively engaged in such a programme. Young girls and women risk death in childbirth as a result of both practices.

The issue of male circumcision was not specifically addressed. It appears to be an accepted practice. However, there may be physical and social consequences. Certainly the intervention is not practised in the most hygienic environment. In some countries, such as Egypt, the implications of the practice for men's sexual health is being explored and challenged.

# Appendix 5
# Case study 3: Ali Roba, Metta, Eastern Hararge

## Background

Ali Roba, the research site, is located in Metta woreda, Eastern Hararge. The majority of the population are Oromo. Metta borders Deder, where the Oxfam regional office is located, and has recently been created a woreda in its own right. The vast majority of people are Muslims. There is a minority Christian population. It is a fertile highland region, which has been of late increasingly given over to growing 'chat, an addictive stimulant used by a majority of the male population, and a smaller number of women. This mass addiction has serious implications for the socio-economic potential in the region and the health status of men in particular. Apart from sales on the local market, 'chat is supplied across the border into Djibouti and Somalia, and farther to Yemen. Fluctuations in the market price for 'chat affect household food security.

Chelenko town, 12km from the site, is the capital of Metta woreda. There is a bustling local market selling livestock, grains, vegetables, fruits, household goods, cloth, and 'chat. The vast majority of traders are women, many trading in 'chat. The population of Metta woreda is 172,803, 96% of them living in rural areas. There are roughly equal numbers of males and females in the woreda, and out-migration did not appear to be a major feature, although some men migrate to Dire Dawa and Harar in search of work.

The region was subjected to the Derg regime's programme of villagisation. Ownership of productive assets such as land and livestock was affected. Households were organised into Peasant Associations (PAs) for the purpose of the co-operative organisation of agricultural production. Men and boys were conscripted into the army, and some women lost their husbands in the civil war that was waged during Mengistu's time. It is in the front line, bordering with Somalia in the east. While the community in the research site was hoping for a quiet life, there was an awareness of the potential for instability due to extremist Oromo Liberation Movements operating in the region. The road leading from Addis to Deder was not safe to travel after 4.00 p.m., and two travellers had been killed on the road two weeks before the research team passed through.

### The site selected for research

Ali Roba, a village some 40km from Deder and 12km from Chelenko, was selected by the Oxfam regional office. It is part of an active PA, whose Chairman assisted the team throughout the ten-day stay. Some households in the village had benefited from Oxfam's Integrated Development Programme (1993–1996), which was now in a consolidation phase in partnership with the Ministry of Agriculture (MoA). The MoA's development agent also assisted the team. Oxfam interventions included water supply, soil and water conservation and re-afforestation, and credit groups for petty trade (mostly women) and livestock ownership, in particular oxen (mostly men). There was also a modern bee-keeping project. The credit programme for women traders was very popular, as was the oxen credit scheme.

Oxfam's involvement in the village gave the team a very positive opening. The women were reluctant to begin with, particularly as they were responsible for feeding their families from their daily income from trade. However, by the end of the PRA, the women were singing and dancing and thanking the team for coming. They had learned a lot about themselves by going through this process.

### Number of people involved in the research

There was a total of 82 participants in the focus groups: two groups of 12 men; two groups of 12 women; two single-sex youth groups of 12, aged 10–18 years; and one group of 10 PA leaders, including one woman, the Chairwoman of the women's wing. In addition, 35 households participated in one-to-one interviews, and 30 were selected for analysis, including eight men and 22 women. More women than men were interviewed, since the process included an in-depth section on women's reproductive-health issues as well as livelihoods, incomes and expenditure, general health problems, and education.

A total of 13 professionals in the education service were interviewed, all men except one woman teacher. These included the Acting Head of the Woreda Education Office; the Director and two teachers, and six members of the PTA at Dudela 3 Elementary School in Ali Roba; and the Director of Chelenko Elementary school.

A total of eight health professionals (all men) were interviewed. These included the Health Service Director of Chelenko Clinic (a health assistant); the Sanitarian for Metta Woreda; the Head of the Woreda Health Bureau; the Manager of the Woreda Environmental Health Department; the General Surgeon and the head nurse at Deder hospital; and two nurses at Chelenko health centre. A total of six traditional practitioners were interviewed, including a (male) Sheik herbalist; two (female) TBAs; one (female) TBA who had been trained 15 years previously; a male Herbalist; and a drug-store owner and traditional health practitioner in Chelenko (male).

## Poverty, nutrition, and livelihoods

Women and men identified the following problems.

- **Agriculture:** *'Our crop was damaged by flood. We lost its harvest and have nothing during this year.'* (Men)
- **Land:** *'Shortage of land for cultivation.'* (Men) *'Land deterioration and lack of money to buy inputs.'* (Men)
- **Water:** Shortage of potable water. (Men and women)
- **Irrigation:** *'We were digging this spring to get some water for irrigation. We need help to dig the stones out.'* (Men)
- **Food:** *'Due to hunger we could not send our children to school.'* (Men). Can't afford to follow nutrition advice for their children. (Women)
- **'Chat:** Depression in the market, and increasing taxes on 'chat, seriously affecting incomes and ability to purchase food. (Men)
- **Health centre:** *'We do not have health centre to take our children for treatment, or to go to when we get sick, even if we have the money.'* (Men) *'We can't get money immediately to take our children to the health centre. By the time we bring the money, the children have died, or become worthless.'* (Women)
- **Medication:** The high cost of medication. (Men)
- **School:** School in the village has Grades 1–4 only. (Men) *'It has enough rooms but has a shortage of teachers. It could be expanded to teach students up to Grade 8.'* (Women)
- **Security:** Worried about *'peace and the safety of our children'.* (Men)
- **Ill health:** *'If you are healthy you can even work as a daily labourer and earn some money.'* (Women)
- **Death of spouse:** *'Loss of partner is a problem for work on the farm.'* (Women)
- **Grinding mill:** *'We travel a long distance to get our grain milled. It takes around two hours' round trip.'* (Women)

The men's group explained that for the majority of households, i.e. the worst-off, the main problem was *'to secure their daily bread'*. They said that poorer women, often widows, were *'worried to find food for their family and always toil, they search for firewood because they only have very small plots of land.'* Women said that *'the problems affect women more. Health problems as well as other problems affect mostly women.'*

### Difficult months

At the time of the research, March 1999, the women and men in Ali Roba reported that the region had been suffering from drought, so there were low incomes and no food. The price for 'chat had dropped significantly, further diminishing the ability to buy food. May to August (Ginbot to Nehasse) were reported as the most difficult months in the year. While men reported high incomes from harvests in July, the women's group and 35% of the worst-off household-heads interviewed (75% of whom were female) reported that July was the worst month for income. This substantiates men's argument that they are in control of the main family income.

### Poverty ranking

The adult focus groups were asked to identify criteria for distinguishing the well-being and poverty of different households. They classified **worst-off households** as those with large families (seven children); or where the spouse, especially the husband, is dead; where women have to bring up children alone; where the mother might have land, but no male help to produce; or she has no livestock; or she is old, sick, or disabled. Men in 'worst-off' households were described as 'chat traders or sellers of firewood; or they did daily labour on other's land. Their land may be too small; they may not produce 'chat; or they may have to share a small area of land with a father or son. They may have to resort to share-cropping.

**Medium-poor households** were defined as those able to send children to school. The head works as a daily labourer, or has land and sells 'chat or firewood; might be a salaried businessman; or might have a small amount of land, and *'he and his wife are strong enough to work'*.

**Better-off households** were defined as those that owned enough land and could grow 'chat and/or have sufficient livestock.

## Factors contributing to increasing poverty

- The drought: it has affected the production of 'chat, grains, and vegetables, and food security.
- Losing access to land, especially 'chat land.
- Becoming a widow, losing a husband's labour (especially ploughing).
- Becoming a widower, losing women's labour, losing trading income, and losing a carer for the household and children.
- Serious health problems which require selling assets or borrowing money to seek treatment.
- Being hungry and physically weak, not having the strength to work.
- Changes in market prices, e.g. the price of 'chat had decreased.

## Signs of increasing poverty

- Breakdown in social customs: sharing food and inviting neighbours does not happen any more (women reporting).
- Land distribution: high incidence of 'accidents' arising from violent disputes within families over land (men and health-service providers reporting).
- Impact of 'chat: few used to chew it in Haile Selassie's time. Addiction has gradually increased until virtually all males over 15 are chewing 'chat (old man reporting, health-service providers' comments, and team observation).
- Women increasing their petty trading in addition to their over-stretched burden in domestic labour and agriculture. Dependency of families on incomes of 3.00 – 5.00 Birr from women's 'chat trade.
- Low incomes and increasing market prices for food commodities.

The health and education service providers were unanimously agreed that the cost of education and health care was too high for the majority, who were in the worst-off households.

## Access to resources and communications

- The nearest health centre is in Chelenko: *'one hour's walk for a healthy person, four hours' walk for a sick one'*. The nearest hospital is 40km away in Deder.
- There is one elementary school in the village, which caters for Grades 1–4. None of the focus-group participants had a child in the elementary school in Chelenko, which covers Grades 5–8.
- There is no market in the village; the nearest is in Chelenko.
- There is a small 'suk' with basic provisions, including some basic medicines.
- There is piped water, installed by the community with Oxfam assistance.
- There are no phones or easy access to transport. Most people walk.
- There are mosques in and around the village for the majority Muslim population, but no church for Christians.
- Women, especially widows, had less access within the village to credit for health costs and education than men did. Men with 'chat fields had the greatest chance of borrowing, but now the 'chat market has dropped in value, even 'chat farmers said it was difficult to borrow. *'Now this hope we lost, nobody lends to the poor.'*

## Social relations

The team gained a strong impression that women and girls in Oromo society were seriously oppressed. Men control the main source of household income and land. They are represented in key organisations which potentially influence the socio-economic and religious lives of the whole community. These include the school committee, the mosque, the Koran school, and the Peasant Association. There was no doubt, however, that for the household economy to function, men need women and their skills and contribution, and women need men's. Women's well-being drops more dramatically than men's on the death or serious illness of their spouses, since it is only men who can plough the land, and it is men who inherit and defend land. There is a serious shortage of land, because of population growth, the inheritance system, and the land-distribution policies that have been implemented in the region. Land is of such crucial importance to survival in the absence of other important sources of livelihood that one of the main health problems reported was accidental injury as a result of feuds between male family members over land.

This was the only site where there were several corroborated reports of physical violence – by men against brothers and fathers over land, by men against wives, and by women and men against children. There were reports of children being regularly whipped and beaten in order to ensure that they grow up properly. Violence was attributed to the effects of 'chat addiction: when the immediate effect wears off, addicts become increasingly unpredictable and aggressive.

## Livelihoods

This is a subsistence-agriculture economy, dependent on the productivity and contribution of all household members of all ages. Men's productivity is influenced by their addiction to 'chat. It appears that there is a significant onus on women to provide, particularly in the most difficult months.

It is important to understand the gender/age division of labour and its connection with the physical and mental burdens which women and girls in particular bear, especially in the context of their reproductive-health status. Their workload, their physical health, and their gender-based reduced access to resources relative to men's seriously undermine their ability to maintain the health and welfare of their children, who are visibly undernourished, dirty, and poorly. Boys' and girls' significant contribution to the household economy reduces time available for school and potentially affects their health status.

There were many products being sold in the market in Chelenko. These included shoes, clothes and traditional shemma (second-hand and new), grains, spices, yam, potato, mango, banana, lemon, onion, garlic, vegetables, handicrafts including pottery and baskets, firewood and charcoal, seeds, tobacco and coffee leaves for hodja tea, and coffee. Many items are produced by the rural population and sold by a large proportion of women and girls, and by some men and boys.

*Men's work*

**Agriculture:** *'Maize, sorghum, barley, potato, yam, sweet potato and 'chat are grown by men. Livestock for dairy production and oxen fattening for sale is done by men.'* Men are responsible for ploughing and preparing the land, including women's vegetable plots. Men did not recognise women's contribution to agriculture; they said, *'Men do it'*. However, women gave detailed descriptions of their work in agriculture.

**Livestock:** Women said that in medium-poor households they *'fatten oxen to sell for a better price'*. They also *'rear sheep for sale in difficult times'*. Money from the sale of livestock *'we use for schooling, health, etc'*. Although women may also be feeding the animals, men generally decide on and control the sale of livestock.

**Men's trading:** Although some men are petty traders like the women, men are more likely to be trading the higher-value items, and in larger quantities. They oversee the sale of livestock and crops. In the market in Chelenko, men were involved in wholesale trading of charcoal and grains.

**Bee-keeping:** *'Ato Selama Husen, one of the very worst-off, earns about 30.00 birr a month from his beehives.'* Improved bee-keeping and training is one of Oxfam's projects in the area.

**Daily labour:** *'Poor men go to far places and do daily labour to generate income for the family.'*

*Women's work*

**Agriculture:** *'We help our husbands on their farmland, weeding and other farm activities.'* They are also involved in hoeing, watering, weeding, husking, and collecting and piling straw for animal feed. They said that they also bring hodja (local tea made with milk) and food, and sing and dance in the fields to encourage the men in their work.

**Horticulture:** *'We grow vegetables and fruit which we sell in the market to earn money and supplement our family diet (especially with sweet potato).'*

**Porterage:** A large part of women's work involved carrying. TBAs linked women's heavy porterage to complaints of pain in the uterus (umbilical hernia). At harvest time, *'Women carry the harvest in a 'debo' [a work group]'*. *'Women carry the soil from the fertile land to the crop land to make the soil more fertile.'* *'Women irrigate the crops and carry them to market.'* During ploughing time, *'The woman prepares hodja and food before she leaves to trade in the market. She feeds the animals, and if the husband needs help, she carries the plough to the field for him.'*

**Petty trade:** About 10–20 women have formed an association ('ekub') in which one woman takes the milk produced by all of them to market. She can use the income immediately. Instead of going to market with a cup of milk every day and earning one or two birr, each woman goes with 20 cups every 20 days or so, and earns a larger sum. Women also sell vegetables and *'njera for those who need to buy'*.

Men sell the 'chat crop if they have a donkey or if a customer comes to the field, '*otherwise when the husband is harvesting ['chat], the woman carries it on her back to the market*'. Many women are 'chat traders: '*Women work hard to keep their families. A [woman] 'chat trader wakes up around 5.00 a.m. to go to another village. She buys 'chat and travels back to Chelenko to sell. There are times when the women get back around 10.00 p.m.*' Small children are left with older sisters. In the household survey, 77% of women from the poorest households reported being engaged in 'chat trade or selling firewood.

**Daily labour:** '*Able bodied, healthy women travel to small towns to earn an income from daily labour.*' They carry and fetch water, clean and wash for households in town.

**Domestic work:** Women and girls are responsible for cooking, cleaning, collecting water and firewood, and caring for children and the sick. They also organise children, both boys and girls, to help. More girls than boys miss school as a result.

*Children's work*
Children's contribution to the household economy is essential and taken for granted. They also need to learn these tasks for adulthood, which, especially for girls, starts all too early.

**Agriculture and livestock:** The women said: '*Boys help their fathers digging (hoeing) and weeding. They also look after the animals.*' '*Girls also look after animals.*'

**Domestic labour:** '*The girls help in the house, they collect water, cook and clean the house. They collect firewood and wash clothes.*' In fact, '*some boys do girls' work and some girls do boys' work, it depends*' – on how many boys and girls there are in the family and how old they are.

**Petty trading:** In Chelenko market, boys were buying quantities of bread rolls to sell at a 75% mark-up. One boy interviewed was paying for his schooling this way. Efitu, a young girl trading to support her family, was selling milk at 2.90 Birr per litre.

## Incomes and expenditures

The household-survey data confirmed that sales of 'chat and other crops were the main sources of income. In 50% of the worst-off households and 71% of the medium households, the main source of income was from 'chat sales. Only 5% of the household-survey respondents reported

sale of livestock as a source of income, and only then as a secondary source. In the focus groups it emerged that livestock is sold only when there is a specific need; men said that they fatten and sell once a year on a Muslim holiday.

With regard to decision-making on expenditures, the men said: '*All expenditures are decided by joint discussion, but most of the time men decide.*' Then they said: '*The money is kept by the women.*' Women said: '*Purchasing cattle is men's decision*', while '*Purchase of household items like food, kerosene, school materials is decided by women.*' In the household survey the majority of worst-off households reported that men control the income, even if women earned it. In the medium households, women were reported to have proportionately greater control over income than in the worst-off group.

In this region, men lie and sit around chewing 'chat, smoking tobacco, and drinking hodja for much of the day. There are seasons when they are active in agriculture; otherwise in general women manage the day-to-day needs of the household.

In the worst-off group, 30% reported earning less than 50.00 Birr per month (US$6.40), even in good times. The women estimated that on average poorer women might earn 2.00 to 5.00 Birr (US$ 0.25 – 0.64) per day, for a family of six. One woman explained: '*My husband is sick. We don't earn an income from land because he can not work on the land. I earn money by trading. With this sort of business I get nothing. The average is 3.00 – 5.00 Birr per day.*'

A slightly better-off woman said: '*I have a husband. We work together on the land. We get around 3 quintals per year. However, I do not sit around the whole day waiting for the crop. I go and sell 'chat in the market. I earn 3.00-10.00 Birr [US$ 0.38 – 1.28] per day. There are days when I do not earn any money. There are days when I even lose the capital I spent on the 'chat.*'

The lowest-income month for 43% of households in the survey was July, followed by August. During these bad months, 60% of worst-off households reported incomes of less than 50.00 Birr ($US 6.40), and at least a third of these households are single-parent families. In medium households which have a small 'chat plot, 71% reported earning less than 100.00 Birr ($US 12.80) per month.

## Food security

At the time of the research, this community was under stress, as a result of poor harvests due to drought and adverse weather conditions over the past two to three years. Signs of malnutrition were visible and were pointed out by participants in the focus groups. These included diseases such as swollen body and diarrhoea, and a significant incidence of miscarriage reported by TBAs.

*Meals per day*

The men said: *'Due to the drought we are not sure to eat once a day.'* In the household interviews it was reported that in difficult months (including the survey period) 43% of boys and 42% of girls, and 54% of men and 53% of women in worst-off households, had one meal per day. In the women's focus group, they said: *'We are eating once a day, and there are days when we go without food for a day or more.'* In 71% of households interviewed, a meal consisted of a handful of roasted cereal ('kollo') such as barley or wheat. Women said of the nutrition advice given by health workers: *'We know that our children should get potatoes mixed with onion and eggs, but we can't afford it.'* Some women wished they could give their own children the milk and eggs that they sell in the market to buy grain.

*Sources of food*

People access food from their own crops and by buying. When they finish their own crop, women sell 'chat to buy food. The shift from food to 'chat production has reduced the availability of food from their own farms. Sweet potato and beans are inter-cropped, and some sorghum is grown, but little else. From a woman's daily earnings of 3.00–5.00 Birr, little can be bought. In the market in Chelenko at the time of the survey, teff was sold at 2.00 Birr per kilo, sorghum at 1.70 per kilo, and maize at 1.60 per kilo. One day's work may buy one and a half kilos of teff for a family of six.

*Expenditure on food*

In the household survey it was reported that 88% of income was spent on food in good months and 94% in bad months. In worst-off households, 30% woman-headed, 95% of income was spent on food in bad months and 89% in good months. In 97% of all households interviewed, difficulty in maintaining adequate nutrition was reported. The local elementary-school teachers confirmed that children did not get enough food. Both professional and traditional health-service providers attributed most health problems to malnutrition and poor sanitation.

## Coping strategies

- *The better-off help the poorest* by hiring them to work on their farms. However, during times of drought there is less work.
- *Trading and daily labour*, especially by women. There was little agricultural labour for men, due to the drought. Women work in domestic labour in town, in fetching water and firewood, and cleaning.
- *Eating under-ripe food*. Some women collect and prepare under-ripe sorghum and vegetables in order to feed their children.
- Some better-off households *sell livestock* when they are short of cash and to pay for health care or schooling.
- *Borrowing money* – although only few reported being able to do so.
- Men are leaving land fallow, and *'we pray to Allah to solve our problem'*.

# Health

There is a new government health centre, opened in March 1999, in Chelenko, about 10km from Ali Roba. The hospital is in Deder, 40km away. There are several TBAs and about four herbalists in the village. People also go to the Muslim Sheiks for healing. The government health staff said that people come for treatment only when the illness is very serious. At Deder hospital most patients are not exempt from fees. In Chelenko they reported that it was mostly men who come for curative care and women who come for preventative treatment. These women, however, appear to be largely the better-off urban dwellers.

The government service providers did not list women's reproductive-health problems as 'main health problems', but the community did. Many procedures relating to these are carried out in the village and/or dealt with outside the government health service. Procedures such as tonsilectomy and uvelectomy are also performed by traditional herbalists.

## Causes of health problems

Health-service providers attributed common health problems to malnutrition, poverty, and poor sanitation. According to men, to Alibaye (a traditional and modern healer in Chelenko), and to nursing staff at the clinic, 'chat was the cause of violent outbursts, resulting in traumatic injury, and of impotence. There was also a high incidence of gonorrhoea, on which men consult

**Table 23: The most common health problems identified by the focus groups**

| Men's group | Women's group | Boys' group | Girls' group | Govt. health-service providers |
|---|---|---|---|---|
| Paralysis | | | Rheumatic pains | |
| TB | TB | TB | | TB, especially pulmonary |
| Diarrhoea | Amoeba/diarrhoea with blood | Intestinal parasites Diarrhoea | Amoeba/diarrhoea With blood | Parasitic diseases, schistoma, hook worm |
| Scabies | Swollen body | | Kidney problems | Skin diseases |
| Effects of 'chat' | Cold/headaches/ Fever | Common cold | Headaches Coughs | Respiratory-tract infection |
| Girls' circumcision | Measles | | Girls' circumcision Early pregnancy & related childbirth problems | Gonorrhoea |
| Accidents –oxen | Tonsilitis | | Gastritis | Gastritis, ulcers |
| Violence: fighting & domestic violence | Excess bleeding (delivery) | | | Accidents caused by homicidal injury |
| Swollen bodies especially children | Swollen bodies especially children | | | Malnutrition/ Anemia |
| | | | | Eye diseases |

traditional herbalists, because they will not get treatment at the health centre unless they bring their partners.

There was insufficient immunisation coverage. Alibaye said that children die of measles as a result, and the health assistants in Chelenko and Deder were far from satisfied with the outreach service. It was under-funded and poorly staffed. In Ali Roba, women seemed to immunise their children if the outreach service came, but 50% of infants in the worst-off households had not been vaccinated. Some women were suspicious and believed that the injection could make their children ill.

'Paralysis' was mentioned in all focus groups and was said to be dealt with by the herbalists. The men's group attributed it to 'chat, which *sucks our blood, that is why we represented paralysis by its leaves*'; but the youth groups reported that everyone suffers from it.

The men's group thought that women got TB by '*carrying heavy loads and by beatings over the back and shoulders*'. Domestic violence, according to

one of the TBAs, does occur, though it is obviously a taboo subject, judging from the conflicting reports. The women's group, for example, said there was no domestic violence.

**Effects of health problems on livelihoods**

Poor health was reported to lead to reductions in family income; reductions in the number of meals eaten per day, affecting all family members; the sacrifice of other activities to look after the sick; and the inability to plough, if the husband was sick. Keeping up with school was important to both boys and girls. Some said that illness kept them away from school. The teachers in Ali Roba reported that diarrhoeal diseases in particular kept children out of school.

**Seasonal patterns**

The surgeon at Deder hospital maintained that hospital records of top ten diseases at any point in time were more a reflection of the community's

91

access to cash to pay for treatment at different times in the year than a reflection of actual patterns of incidence. There were, however, some distinct patterns, such as border disputes and resultant traumatic injury, increasing during the dry season when men are irrigating their land. Many problems reportedly occurred throughout the year: women's health problems, parasites, paralysis, scabies, and malnutrition-related illnesses such as swollen body in children.

The hot dry season, April to June, saw food shortages, low incomes, and a high prevalence of diarrhoeal diseases, according to the men's group and Alibaye, the healer in Chelenko. He said that people have no latrines, and faeces are all over the place, spreading disease. The rainy season also brought a high incidence of diarrhoea, because of faecal contamination of the drinking water (in Deder).

The woreda health office reported a higher incidence of gonorrhoea during the 'chat harvest season, July and August, when men get high on 'chat; some, he said, have a high sexual drive, others become impotent.

### Reproductive-health issues

Many reproductive-health conditions, rituals, and problems were dealt with in the village by traditional herbalists or untrained birth attendants. These included male circumcision, female genital mutilation, treatments for impotence and gonorrhoea, childbirth, and pregnancy-related problems. Women tended to use services if they came as outreach.

**Family planning:** Here, as in Somali region, it was seen as important to have large families. In the worst-off households interviewed, 90% said they were not using family planning, mostly because they wanted more children. Only 4% said they were not aware of family-planning methods, and they were all in the worst-off households. The large number of children was seen as a problem by men only in the context of land shortage and inheritance rights, and by parents because they could not afford to send so many to school.

**Circumcision:** All girls and boys are circumcised, girls when they are between 5 and 7 years, and some later at 12 or 13 years old. The most extreme form of FGM, infibulation, is practised in Ali Roba. The clitoris is removed, as are the labia minora and labia majora. The wound is stitched to leave a tiny opening for urine and menstrual flow. The girls' group knew

that '*it is not good to circumcise girls*'. They wanted to know more about FGM and its hazards. They did not really know why it should be performed, except that it had always been done. Health education advising against FGM has obviously filtered through to Ali Roba. However, although the men's group included FGM among one of the most common health problems, they said: '*We don't believe anything that is said on the mass media ... about the negative consequences of girls' circumcision*'. On the contrary, women said such things as: '*I do not know anyone until now who is not circumcised, and who did not have a problem during delivery. The TBAs operate with a blade, and there will be excess bleeding.*' FGM, according to the surgeon in Deder hospital, can cause obstructed birth, a ruptured bladder, and incontinence thereafter. However, all girls continue to be circumcised, and there were no signs of action to change attitudes to girls' sexuality and reproductive rights, nor to eliminate the practice.

**Antenatal care:** ANC attendance at the old Chelenko clinic was low and declining. In Ali Roba, 52% of women in the household interviews had not used ANC in their last pregnancy. In the worst-off category, 70% of those who had sought ANC had visited the outreach service when it came. On average, those who attended ANC reported attending one to three times during their pregnancy. Almost one-third of women complained of problems during their most recent pregnancy.

**Early marriage, early pregnancy, and childbirth:** Early marriage and early pregnancy are common. The boys, when asked what health education they would like to pass on to their parents, included '*the prevention of early marriage*'. The Chairwoman of the women's wing of the PA accused the Chairman of the PA and other PA leaders of not doing enough to stop early marriage. She thought the PA and the schools should work closely together, particularly to persuade parents on this issue.

Not one woman in the household interviews had been attended by a trained medical person during her most recent delivery. All had given birth at home, 93% with an untrained traditional birth attendant, the remainder with the one, trained, birth attendant in the village. She, however, has had no training in over 15 years, is not supervised, and has no kit. TBAs wanted training and kits and contact with the health centre. The health centre had a programme to train TBAs, but Ali Roba was not included. Given the huge demand, the response is limited, largely because of inadequate funds and staffing. Dr Tekolla, surgeon at Deder hospital, confirmed that the number of women attended by a medical professional in childbirth was negligible. The main problem reported by women was excess bleeding after delivery. Women attributed it to poor nutrition, and some, they said, die unless they get some fatty foods.

## Quality and affordability of health care

The main criteria that people used for judging quality included cost; cleanliness; availability of diagnostic and other equipment; the attitude of the medical staff; waiting times; cure rates; and drug availability.

The government health services are too expensive for people in Ali Roba. They go only when the problem is severe and if they manage to borrow money. The poorest, and women in particular, have difficulty in accessing credit. In households interviewed, 75% said that health services were unaffordable or only affordable with a struggle. For them, the cost of health care is not just the fees. Women included costs such as transport and food and accommodation for the treatment of TB patients in Deder hospital. Similarly, women could not afford the 'treatment' advised for their malnourished infants. Women's access to good food to feed the family appeared to be central to maintaining health and to preventing many of the main health problems, but they cannot afford to adopt the advice that they are given.

All focus groups, the youth in particular, were scathing about traditional herbalists and healers, largely because of the cost and the slim chance of a cure. Boys said they lack the knowledge and medicine, girls said they make people crazy and are not effective.

The women and girls in particular had great faith in Alibaye, the traditional and modern-medicine drug-store owner in Chelenko. However, medication in both government facilities and at Alibaye's was too expensive. Several women said that they just go to the kiosk in the village to get some painkillers. The government medical professionals agreed that there was a shortage of medication. Some of the medication supplied was not required, and some ran out within two months of delivery, leaving the health facility with nothing for months. Medication was too expensive for most people.

The surgeon, Dr Tekolla, also had an excellent reputation with the people. The main problem with government facilities was the cost and the waiting time. This is crucial, since people do not seek treatment until their condition is already very critical. The women said: 'People can die waiting.'

The majority of women reported that the untrained TBAs were very dirty. The only birth attendant who was respected was the trained birth attendant.

Government health professionals said that there was a shortage of funds and staff for effective running of the immunisation, FP, ANC, family health, and health-education programmes, both on-site and outreach. They believed that outreach was immensely important, to help them to work more closely with the community, particularly on the prevention of diseases and on family planning.

Generally, men are not targeted by the family health programme, FP education, etc. Given their position of power and control in the community and the enormity of women's reproductive-health problems, this may be a serious oversight.

## Source of money for health care

Most households reported that people borrowed money if they could, or sold livestock or household assets. Not all families were in a position to do any of these: 'The only option we have is to wait on a bed to die.' While the women's group did not know very much about the exemption system or how it worked, the men were relatively well informed.

# Education

Participants said that there had been a shift in opinion about education, especially since the Derg's period. In Haile Selassie's time it used not to be valued at all, and only boys, if anyone at all, were sent to school. Now the underlying problem was poverty: the lack of income, and the fact that children's labour is integral to the household economy. Girls were needed for domestic labour and to produce baskets for sale in the market, boys were needed to look after livestock. In the market survey it was noted that quite a number of traders were school-age girls, some of whom were illiterate.

Children in Ali Roba have three options for elementary schooling: Dudela No. 3 Elementary School (Grades 1–4) in Ali Roba; Dudela No. 4 (Grades 1–4); and the Chelenko Elementary and Junior Secondary School (Grades 1–8). Most of the children who go to school attend the elementary school in Ali Roba. All participants wanted the grades to be extended at least to Grade 6. No one in the focus groups had a child attending school in Chelenko: it was just too distant. There was also a Koran school in the village.

Despite women and men in the focus groups saying that education is equally valuable for both girls and boys, very few of either sex go to school, and proportionately even fewer girls are sent. Education-service providers estimated that about 65% of all children do not go to school, and that 75% of girls do not attend. In the household interviews (where 73% of respondents were women), 43% said there was no advantage to educating boys, and 57% no advantage to educating girls. There is still a problem of attitude to education, particularly among an adult population which is largely illiterate, or barely literate.

In the worst-off households interviewed, 78% of females of school age and above were illiterate, and 31% of males. While only 24% of males had attended elementary education between Grades 1 and 4, a mere 2% of females had. In Dudela Elementary school in Ali Roba (Grades 1–4), some classes had only 3% girls attending. Exposure to education was abysmally low, and for women and girls even lower than for their male counterparts. Another issue mentioned was that children start school relatively late. The average age in Grade 1 was 9 years old.

Teachers said that girls' performance in school was worse than boys'. This was attributed to the culture and the fact that girls are brought up to be shy and withdrawn and boys to be outgoing. Girls, they said, also had domestic work to do before and after school. Other factors inhibiting girls' attendance included early marriage and early pregnancy. Early marriage also affected boys' school attendance, but whereas boys might enter marriage at 18, girls can get married at 12 or 13 years. The men also reported that girls can spend up to three months recovering from FGM; this will also affect their access to school.

Education was considered to be unaffordable, particularly for the worst-off households (the majority), by participants and service providers. The cost of schooling was considered to include the cost of food, clothing, cleanliness, and school materials like exercise books and pens. All this was unaffordable. One woman said: *'We send only boys to school, because of lack of enough money to send both children to school. If we keep girls at home, they produce woven baskets, which they take to the market to sell. That will enable the family to send the boys to school.'*

The main reasons for non-attendance or dropping out of school were given by education-service providers as follows: many schools are too far away from where children are living; girls are victims of customs and religion; girls get married at an early age; girls are not encouraged to go to school; many parents have low levels of awareness regarding the value of education; girls are wanted to help at home; boys are needed to tend animals; more boys drop out because they are involved in petty trade, mainly selling 'chat; parents could not afford clothing and school supplies; the school [in Chelenko] is full to capacity and overcrowded. In general there was an agreement that *'in most cases, the children of the worst-off groups are the main victims'*.

The school PTA said that children did not attend school because of parental poverty; the shortage of teachers at the school; the lack of money to buy pens and exercise books; and diseases such as diarrhoea.

There was a high drop-out rate reported by service providers. The class size in Grade 1 was typically much larger than that in Grade 4. In the school in Ali Roba, for example, the 1989 Grade 1 intake had fallen by 41% over the two years to 1991. The largest number of drop-outs was among boys, linked to the fact that boys make up the larger proportion of children in school. Boys drop out in order to work or trade during the worst months of the year.

The schools suffer from a lack of textbooks: one book is shared between two to five children. Teachers do not have teacher's guides, and the courses translated into Orominya from Amharic are often too difficult for the students. Some teachers are reportedly under-qualified for the grades they are teaching and do not understand the material either. There are not enough adequately qualified teachers. Teachers think that, for the hours they work, the conditions and the cost of living, their salaries are inadequate.

There was a shortage of desks and chairs, and no water in school compounds. Many have no toilets, though there was one at the school in Ali Roba. In general, while the demand for services from an increasingly impoverished and growing population increases, it appears that funding for education materials, medication, staffing and staff training, equipment, and proper sanitation is totally inadequate to cope. Neither the schools nor the health centre receive any cash budget of their own to cover costs. Salaries are paid for by the woreda offices, and materials and medication are received in kind. The staff who manage these services have no control whatsoever over their supply. Assistance from donors has to be applied for through the woreda office, which decides on the distribution of materials among the various facilities. The UNICEF WIBS programme provides some school furniture and funds some short workshops for teachers, but in the face of the demand this is a drop in the ocean.

Both education and health-care personnel have a very tough existence in this remote area. They lack training to upgrade themselves and they lack access to libraries and entertainment facilities. A woman teacher said that work was difficult without child-care support for her two small children, and the distance to market without transport made provisioning difficult.

It has to be said that the research team was enormously impressed by the dedication to their work and to the people that was demonstrated by many of the service providers interviewed, including the translators from the health service and MoA who worked with us.

# Appendix 6
# Case study 4: Belhare, Jijiga, Somali Region

In Sheik Umer, the men told the researchers: '*If you had come before the problem, you could have helped. Now the problem has already cost the lives of our cattle.*' The men said there was a need for fundamental change: '*We always discuss problems after they have taken place. There should be some serious planning to* prevent *problems.*'

## Introduction

The woreda of Jijiga is located in Somali Region, bordering Somalia. It is physically and psychologically remote. The region is accessed by the road from Harar between the 'safe' hours of 9.00 a.m. and 1.00 p.m. At other times, travellers risk being accosted by 'shiftas' or bandits from one or other of the more extremist Somali clans. The area is associated with contraband trade, including the stimulant drug 'chat.' The people have suffered drought and war, and signs of the latter are still visible in the form of derelict tanks scattered over the wide open plains, or at the edge of a village.

The population in the woreda as a whole is 248,465, according to the 1994 census, 74% of whom live in the rural areas. The rural population is characterised by nomadic customs and traditions; men have control over decision-making and the livestock, and women have the main responsibility for the family and domestic sphere, build houses, and care for the smaller ruminants such as goats and sheep. Men dominate the clan structures which shape social and political relations and alliances. Some families have now settled in villages and live as agro-pastoralists, tending livestock and growing food crops.

### Sites selected for research

The two villages visited for the research in March 1999, Sheik Umar and Belhare, are both in Jijiga woreda. They have been settled for over 100 years. After a year with little or no rain, the woreda was seriously affected by drought and food shortage at the time of the research. In both villages livestock were dying, and people had little left to eat or exchange for food. Oxfam Jijiga had already made requests on behalf of the Jijiga DPPB to the Oxfam office in Addis for food aid.

The original site selected for the research was Sheik Umar, a village some 60km east of Jijiga town. No participatory research (PRA) had previously been conducted in the site. It is a recently selected Oxfam project site and has a health committee, organised by the Elders and Oxfam staff. The team spent about a day and a half on the site, conducting the mapping (with women and men), ranking, and seasonal calendars (separate groups of women and men). On the first day of the research the rains started. On the second day there were torrential rains. It took the team three hours to reach the site and four and a half to return to Jijiga. For security reasons it is not advisable to be outside Jijiga town after 5.00 p.m. On the second day the team returned after 7.00 p.m. It was apparent that seven hours of driving limited the time available for research, and it was agreed that in view of security problems the team should look for an alternative site. Belhare village, one of a settlement of five villages 10km outside Jijiga town, was selected.

The people of Belhare are from the Somali ethnic group and speak Somali. They are Muslim and have Koran schools in or near the village. They are not represented by a Peasant Association (PA), the lowest local-level government administrative body which provides a link for development work and provision of services with local woreda authorities in the town. The village belongs to a group of four or five other villages of the same main clan grouping, the 'Akisha', all similarly isolated from official structures and services. The bulk of this report refers to the findings in Belhare village, comprising about 170 households. There were five main sub-clans in Belhare: Hrer Adawi, Werro Sengu, Hrer Tukali, Hrer Ali Boch, and Werro Hamo. Another four clans in the village were Gerri, Charso, Gethe Bursi, and Yebarrhe; these are minority clans and are possibly under-represented and have fewer rights.

Clan loyalty and affiliations underpin social and gender relations and are the source of tensions which can lead to armed conflict. One of the most important social institutions described by the Elders and respected women of Belhare was the 'Hodeyashi Nabadota' (see 'Social relations' below). This is a council of Elders (all men), representing the villages of Belhare, Kordere, Musle, Elbehay, and 'Kaboorelay. The Elders' main function is to maintain the peace. The research does not specifically focus on differentials in access to resources and representation within and between clans and sub-clans, although this is a fundamentally important feature. Work in Somali Region requires a solid understanding of clan structures and dynamics, which influence access to resources and connections at all levels up to regional government.

### Social relations and reproductive health

The team's overall impression of Somali culture was of a community whose survival depends on staying close and sharing resources. Women and men have very distinct and separate spheres. In this system men dominate all decision-making. Women are conditioned from childhood to be retiring and modest, and undertake very specific tasks and responsibilities tied closely to reproduction and home-keeping. They also contribute their labour to agriculture and livestock, but have little or no control over the production output. Having large families is considered important, particularly in this subsistence economy, where everyone's labour contribution counts.

Girls are circumcised and stitched *'to protect them from the boys'* and kept on a tight rein. Without circumcision, girls would be called loose and would never be married. Sexual and reproductive relations, which are also power and control relations, impact significantly on wider social and political relations between women and men and impinge on the representation of women in local and official institutions, where the distribution of resources and power is centralised.

### Number of people involved in the research

In Belhare 24 men and 24 women, and 12 girls and 12 boys (10–18 years) participated in the PRA, and a further 16 women and men took part in a group discussion (Venn diagram) on social institutions. The household survey included 30 interviews: 73% of the respondents were women, and women headed 17% of the households. A significant proportion of questions referred to reproductive health. A total of ten education-service providers were interviewed, including the village Koran school teachers, and five elementary-school teachers in Jijiga. Five interviews were held with health-service providers, including two with TBAs, who were also involved in assisting in female infibulation and the ceremony of cutting a girl, ready for sexual intercourse on her marriage day. Representatives of the Zonal and Regional education and health offices were also interviewed.

## Poverty, nutrition, and livelihoods

### Poverty

The research took place during March, identified by the women in particular as one of the most difficult months each year. This year it was worse, because of the drought. The last crop was harvested over a year ago. The rains needed for ploughing and planting this year's Belg crop were not forthcoming. They had no food crops in store or to sell, and the carcasses of dead animals lay scattered in and around the village.

The drought had completely disrupted the usual rhythm of life and demonstrated to both women and men how dependent they are on the rain for survival, and how vulnerable they are without education. The women's group told us: *'All our hope for the better life depends on the rain which gives us grass and water for our animals, and food production for household consumption.'* The men's group said: *'The effect of drought is that animals are dying, and to live we also sell them. Due to the animals' death and no food, we became weak and get dizzy and we too will die. The children's bodies swell, they get diarrhoea and die or become sick.'*

Throughout the PRA, both the women's and men's groups referred to the low educational status in the community, which denied them a source of leadership and the means to define new strategies to cope with the acute situation created by the drought and the lack of income-generating alternatives.

**Table 24: The main problems identified by women and men in Belhare**

| Main problems | Women | Men |
|---|---|---|
| Transportation/communication | * | * |
| Lack of school in the community | * | * |
| School in Jijiga too far for our children | * | |
| Water: *'all animals including hyena drink with us'* | * | |
| Lack of health service | * | * |
| Lack of ANC | * | |
| Lack of help for pregnant women if there is a problem | * | |
| Lack of food during pregnancy | * | |
| No training for TBAs | * | |
| No delivery materials for TBAs | * | |
| Two years of drought, no rain | | * |
| Animals are dying | | * |
| Disease among people is spreading | | * |

(Source: women and men's focus groups)

## Access to resources and communications

- Belhare has no PA to represent local people or act as a vehicle for development initiatives or provide access to health care via exemption papers.
- There is no clinic; the nearest is 12–15km away. There are no health posts, trained TBAs, or traditional 'bonesetters' (traditional physiotherapists who also provide other therapies) in Belhare itself. The women placed five TBAs on the village map.
- There is no elementary school; the nearest is 12km away. There is a Koran school near the mosque in the village.
- There is no market in Belhare. The villagers go to Jijiga to buy and sell their goods.
- There are no transportation services. People just walk wherever they have to go.

## Poverty ranking

The participants identified 80 households for the ranking, about 47% of the population of Belhare. In 30% of these households, a husband or wife had died. Of these, only four were elderly, 16 were younger men who had died, and three were younger women, leaving growing families behind.

Wealth was ranked according to the number of livestock; the worst-off households, the majority, have no livestock left at all. Shocks such as the loss of a crop, the death of animals, and the death of a spouse all made a household poorer, the men said. Drought had reduced most households to the same level of poverty. When better-off households lose their cattle, not only do they become poorer, but those who depended on their custom lose their source of income too.

Men also said that *'lack of education leads to poverty'*, and that *'health problems make a person poorer'*. The women said that *'life is worse than a few years ago. The problems of school, and water, we know from before. But now the drought makes life worse. There is no food at home for our children and us. Most of the people got sick and died.'* Both the Jijiga Zone Health Bureau and the Region 5 Education Office confirmed that *'people were becoming poorer and poorer, day by day'*.

## Livelihoods

Food crops like maize and sorghum, and livestock including cattle, oxen, camel, sheep, and some goats, form the basis of the subsistence economy. Men reported that they were largely responsible for crops and livestock, and that men control the sale and income from these activities. They said that older boys worked with them in the fields, and women brought the tea. In the household interviews, 71% reported that men control the main source of income, and two-thirds that men either control or share control of the household's secondary income (often women's income) with women.

According to women's reports, however, women were very much involved in agricultural activities, as were girls. Women were also involved in tending livestock and looking for food for animals during the dry season. Although both women and men milk the cows, it was women in Belhare who reported organising themselves into groups for the collection and sale of milk in exchange for grain. (In Sheik Umer, men – not women – sold milk and milk products. Men said the market was too far for women to go. However, women heads of household go to the market in Hartshek.)

Women and girls were largely responsible for all domestic work, including building and maintaining their houses, collecting fuel and water, food processing and preparation, and child care. With marriage and childbirth at 15 not uncommon, girls are forced into adult responsibilities at an early age.

Men reported the months of April and May and from November to January as the most labour-intensive months for agriculture. In normal years, low food availability was reported from April through to September. The worst months for livestock disease and fodder shortage were February and March.

## Incomes

Women and men differed in their assessments of the times of the year for higher incomes. Women clearly had little access to incomes from agriculture. They reported a slight increase in income from August to January, when there is usually an increase in milk production. Men's highest-income months were in the post-harvest months of February and March, income which they spent on agricultural inputs, renting machinery, and buying 'chat and tea to invigorate them for the next round of work in the fields. These months were reported by women to be hard, low-income months. In the household survey, where 73% of respondents were women, March was identified as the worst month in the year for income. This was so in 38% of worst-off, 29% of medium, and 50% of better-off households; 38% of worst-off households reported all year as being bad. During the worst months in the year – and it can be assumed that, for many, the past year had mostly been bad – 83% of all households reported earning less than 50.00 Birr per month ($6.40). However, some reported that they were living on nothing, by begging from neighbours.

Households are relatively large. In Somali society, having many children is still seen as a sign of wealth. In the 'worst-off' category, households averaged six family members. But women in Belhare did classify 'many small children to feed, especially during the drought' as a factor which could contribute to increased poverty.

A strong indicator that this community has few alternative sources of income was the extraordinary proportion of households which reported household members 'doing nothing' during the worst months. In worst-off households, for example, 43% of men, 33% of women, 95% of girls, and 95% of boys were reported to have no income-generating coping strategies to deal with the very bad months in the year.

## Food security

Overall, 70% of respondents reported a dependence on the market for their staple foods. In worst-off households, 90% of income is spent on food during bad months, when incomes were reported to be $3.58 per month. A lower proportion of average incomes was spent on food in good months, when many households, among them even the very poor, had access to some food from their own harvest, or in the form of exchange with and gifts from relatives and neighbours.

The laws of supply and demand, however, mean that grain prices go up when the poor can least afford it. A market survey conducted by the team in Jijiga showed that the price of wheat had increased from 180.00 Birr per quintal to 240.00 Birr in three months, owing to a shortage since the drought. The grain prices from petty traders had increased 100%. At the same time, for those needing to sell smaller livestock to buy food, there had been a downward shift in the prices because of a glut in the market.

Household food consumption has dropped: 100% of households interviewed reported that they were having difficulty in maintaining adequate nutrition for the whole family, because of the drought. At least 52% of all households reported that their children were suffering from malnutrition. The number of children aged 1–15 years in all households totalled 128. Of these, 27% were reported to be suffering the symptoms of malnutrition. In the under-five category, a total of 46 in the households interviewed, 35% were suffering from the symptoms that participants associated with malnutrition. The figures show more boys than girls suffering from malnutrition.

In quite a number of the 80 households ranked, the youngest child was aged 8 years and above. This possibly indicates a high incidence of infant mortality, and/or of malnutrition-related miscarriage. The men's focus group reported that *the main problems are diarrhoea, TB, constipation and getting very weak*. They said that *the children's bodies swell, they get diarrhoea and die or become very sick. The problems got worse over the last three years due to total absence of rain.* According to men, *Children and women are most threatened by the problem.*

One of the TBAs interviewed in Belhare, also responsible for cutting young girls/women on their marriage day, confirmed the increased number of starvation-related illnesses and deaths: *In the last two years lots of people have died, when compared with other times. It is because of starvation.*

### Water and sanitation

The community had no access to clean water: they use open sources, which they share with livestock and wild animals. The women said that *when there was rain, the first dirty water [stagnant] was washed out and we could get the clean water. But now there is no rain, there is a shortage of water to wash away the dirty water.* In the household survey, 100% of households reported collecting water from an open pond, well, or spring for household consumption. It is mostly women and girls who collect water. Men and boys from the worst-off and medium households sometimes collect water in the dry season, when long distances are involved in the search for water.

# Health

There is no clinic within 12km of Belhare. People reported going to the hospital in Jijiga only when their problem was really serious. The household survey and all focus groups indicated strongly that in fact most people stayed at home and prayed to Allah. A few used traditional healers, but recourse to them, apart from for circumcision and childbirth, appeared relatively less common than, for example, in Delanta.

Men appear to be the key decision-makers regarding health-care choices, especially if money is involved. While the girls' focus group said that both mothers and fathers decide on health treatment, the boys were very clear that *the father decides if the treatment requires hospital management; otherwise the mother decides in the case*

*of traditional treatment'*. The men's and women's groups also said that *the husband decides about spending money on health'. 'We call a holy person who knows the Koran to pray for Allah. There is no traditional medicine.'*

In general, participants in the research from the community, and health-service providers, attributed most health problems to poverty resulting from the drought. All prevalent diseases were linked to the lack of adequate nourishment, and to drinking dirty contaminated water. The most common illnesses included diarrhoea, diarrhoea with blood and vomiting, cough, cough and fever, malnutrition, parasites and worms and abdominal swelling, anaemia, excessive bleeding at childbirth, measles, and eye infections. The clinic in El-hamar 12km away provided a very similar profile of the most common illnesses. The problems are widespread.

Médecins sans Frontières Belgium is running a pilot TB programme in Jijiga within the National TB and Leprosy Control Programme. It estimates that 90% of the population is infected with TB (in the sense of having been exposed to it and having their own immunity to it), *but only get sick when they are malnourished, get measles, malaria, whooping cough, or HIV/AIDS'*. It estimated that about 20% of TB patients were HIV-positive, and that 40% of patients admitted to the hospital in Jijiga were HIV-positive.

During the research, the team came to the conclusion that the concept of sickness in a community whose health status is very poor, and which has little or no access to medical treatment, is quite different from that of those who have regular and easy access to health care. Fatuma Arebe, for example, a household-survey respondent, was visibly unwell. She was starving; she and her children all had bloody diarrhoea. Yet she said that she considered herself sick only if she was in bed, and she was not in bed yet. She did not believe you could find a 'free' health service anywhere.

Without a PA, no one in Belhare or the surrounding villages has access to exemption papers. Only a minority in this community, the few remaining better-off households, can 'choose' where they want to go for health care. We repeatedly heard that people just *'get sick and die'*. The boys' group summed up the situation: *Those who have money go to Jijiga hospital. The rest simply stay home and pray for Allah. However, it is only a few who go to Jijiga or visit traditional healers.'* The women's group said: *'We don't know the quality [of govt. services], because we don't go to hospital since we have no money.'*

100

Those who had used the hospital felt discriminated against because of their poverty, dirt, and illiteracy. The men said that the reception of rural patients was not good: 'They like to treat those coming from town, considering them as cleaner.' According to one male participant, 'The poor can only wish.' The cost of treatment and medicine is so high that unless poor people have some relatives to support them, they simply do not go anywhere to get treatment.

The cost of health is also the cost of staying healthy, or of regaining health through good nutrition with medical supervision. Both require assets in livestock, crops and/or cash, and depend on healthy livelihoods. The men's group recounted the story of Mohamed Farah: 'He was sick with diarrhoea last year, and he got anaemia, he did not get treatment. Finally he sold his cow and was admitted to hospital for two months' treatment. It was good treatment, but he is hungry, he is still weak and hungry.'

The problem of mental health is rarely addressed in rural communities. There were some extreme cases cited, including a woman who had three mentally ill children 'tied up at home'. But there were more common signs of mental discomfort pervading all sites in all age groups, linked to a strong sense of insecurity about the future, a fear of starvation, a sense of failure, especially among men, and a sense of real fear and sadness among women when faced with crying, hungry children.

## Women's reproductive health

Women's reproductive-health status is defined by the fact that they are subjected to the most severe form of female genital mutilation at the age of 9–12 years. The report contains a detailed description of the procedure, and subsequent procedures to open the girl at marriage and during childbirth. In this context it is even more deplorable that girls and women do not have access to ANC, nor to any medically qualified person during childbirth.

All women and girls deliver at home: 100% of respondents replied that the place of their most recent delivery was at home. In 93% of households interviewed, an untrained TBA attended the most recent birth. It was telling that, when women were asked questions about poverty during the focus-group discussion, they started talking about the problems they experience during pregnancy and childbirth.

The health assistant at the El-Hamar clinic said that they had no links with TBAs: 'The link we had with TBAs was discontinued when the supply of dry rations they were given as incentives by MSF Belgium was discontinued.' TBAs generally receive no payment from their clients: 'I am not paid a cent. In fact I come home and wash my hands and soiled dress with my own soap. I even walk all the way to Jijiga to buy pain-relieving medicines.'

There is a high fertility rate in this community. Having many children is traditionally welcomed, and women start having children from the age of 15 years or younger. Some women, therefore, responded that even if there were family-planning support, they would not use it. Others reported not using family planning due to lack of knowledge or lack of services.

Women reported not being able to accept hospitalisation of sick children because there was no one to care for their small children at home. The demands of child care, in addition to all the other daily domestic responsibilities, are also most likely to add to a woman's reluctance to prioritise her own health-care needs – particularly reproductive-health problems, since these are taboo.

In Sheik Umer, the men said that women were suffering from malnutrition, and 'unless it is brought by Allah, women do not have other problems'. They considered women's gynaecological problems as 'Allah's or God's will for women'. They said, 'The women do not talk about gynaecological problems. They are shy. Even if they are sick they do not tell men about their diseases, because there are no health-care institutions. They are afraid to talk about these problems.'

## Health-service provision

The Health Bureau reported: 'There is high shortage of equipment, even of materials as inexpensive as pairs of scissors. The hospital has only one microscope, which can only operate when there's electricity. There's a shortage of dressing materials, operation and delivery sets. The shortage of equipment has been exacerbated because old ones became out of use and there is no replacement.'

According to the Zone Health Bureau, 'There is no essential drugs policy. There is severe shortage of drugs in the hospital, health centre and clinics except for niclosomidl and vermox. There is high demand for antibiotics, anti-pain and infusions, which we are extremely short of.' These problems could be solved if the clinic staff were involved in planning and budgeting with the Zonal Department of Health. There is a delay in the release of the budget in general. The budget has continued to decline, except the hospital budget, despite the continuing increase in the number of patients.

The El-Hamar clinic has no knowledge of the budget allocation; in fact, they were puzzled that they had faced some drug shortage that year for the first time in the three years. The clinic is involved in the planning activities and not in the drawing up and allocating of the budget. This is the responsibility of the zonal health department.

At El-Hamar clinic there was reported to be a significant shortage of funds on practically every budget line: drugs, medical equipment, stationery, cleaning materials, and even linen to supply health professionals with the appropriate working uniform. The head of the clinic reported that staff at the clinic have been obliged to use their own bars of soap and powdered soap to wash the reusable syringes and surgical instruments.

The zonal deputy head also mentioned that the World Food Programme provides food supplements at times (supplementary feeding programmes for children). However, he resented the fact that the 'donation' generally arrives within a few days of the expiry date on the food item.

## Immunisation

In all, 40 of the 48 under-fives (83 %) had no access to any type of immunisation. An additional 10%, five children, have defaulted, not because mothers did not want to continue, but because the service was no longer there. Considering the prevalence of measles and TB in the area, in the context of prevailing levels of malnutrition the importance of immunisation to protect this very high-risk and most vulnerable group cannot be over-emphasised. One epidemic of measles could have a disastrous effect, if introduced into this fertile atmosphere of unprotected and malnourished children.

## Education

When asked what actions their families could take to respond to lack of income and production, the women said: '*There is nothing they could do because no one is educated in this area.*' Only five boys from the whole village go to school in Jijiga, 12km away. More boys than girls attend Koran school. The women said: '*Our children tell us what is in the Koran after learning their lesson. The boys come home to tell their sisters and mother about it.*' All lessons are in Arabic, and literacy and numeracy are not taught. The education of girls is controversial, some

fathers noting the need for them to be kept apart from strange boys and men.

In effect, 79% of boys/men in the poorest households were illiterate, and 98% of girls/women; the illiteracy is disempowering and isolates them from the formal government and non-government administrative and service-providing structures. '*No one is educated among us who could lead us,*' the men's group declared. Both women and men thought that if their children were educated they could represent their problems to the appropriate authorities when they were older: '*If our children [boys and girls] were educated, we would not be like this.*' All focus groups also linked education with access to jobs, largely in government employment.

Although there were mostly positive responses about education during the focus-group discussions, the household survey showed that there was some resistance. At least 50% of all respondents (mostly women) did not see the advantage of educating either boys or girls. The youth groups said that many of their parents did not appreciate the value of education. The men said that '*Women do not think about health and education. They only think about how to get food and how to survive.*' They said: '*Women do not even know the Koran, they have no time and are afraid to learn. There is no separate place [from men] for them [to learn the Koran]. They just care for the house, for the children and husband.*'

Access to food, clean water, clothing, and income was identified by the adult focus groups as necessary to sending children to school. Children's labour is an integral part of the household economy. During peak agricultural seasons, demands on boys' labour increase, thus potentially compromising their access to school. Throughout the year, women need their daughters to help them at home and in their productive work. In any case, with such large families, the men said that a family might be able to send only two out of five or seven children to school. Most girls marry and have children early, and this would also interfere with their completing school.

In the region as a whole it was estimated that up to 88% of children were not attending school. One of the reasons given was the lack of classrooms and schools to accommodate all the children. The elementary school visited in Jijiga experienced similar problems to those found in the other sites: lack of textbooks and teaching materials, lack of chairs and desks, no furniture for teachers, no water or toilet facilities, lack of sports facilities, overcrowded classrooms, etc.

Teachers lacked motivation, because of low salaries. There were also problems in attracting teachers who could work and live in such remote areas. Lacking transport, the local authorities were unable to provide the supervision and support necessary.

The 1994 rural population census for Somali region showed that girls/women made up 26% of those currently attending school, and 21% of those who recorded having attended school in the past. The process of socialisation, the burden of domestic and productive work, the expressed need to maintain a separate space for girls, together with circumcision practices and early marriage, certainly inhibit girls from gaining equal access to a complete elementary education.

Education-service providers felt that the potential quality of education was seriously compromised by the lack of necessary materials, equipment, and infrastructure. Teachers' dissatisfaction and the condition of poverty and hunger in which children currently find themselves did not help. For children in and around Jijiga, the Regional Education Bureau said that education *'is too expensive especially for those who have many children'*. At the time of the research they reported that *'drought compels that schools are closed down'*.

www.ingramcontent.com/pod-product-compliance
Lightning Source LLC
Chambersburg PA
CBHW080900030426
42334CB00021B/2612